David Hawker was born in Surrey and educated at Kingston Grammar School. He studied Medicine in Edinburgh, where he met his wife, Beryl, who is also a doctor. He then specialised in Anaesthetics before working in both mission and government hospitals in Pokhara, Nepal for nine years, bringing up their three children there. Returning to the UK, he worked as a GP in Cornwall for 18 years, then on the Hebridean islands of Islay and Jura. He played, and then umpired cricket for 60 years, and loves travel and trains. He has 11 grandchildren. His first book *Kanchi Doctor* was the biography of one of Nepal's first surgeons.

To the resilient people of poverty-stricken rural Nepal and those who seek to help them

David Hawker, Ellen Findlay and
Mike Smith

# MEDICINE IN THE MOUNTAINS

AUSTIN MACAULEY PUBLISHERS™

LONDON ∗ CAMBRIDGE ∗ NEW YORK ∗ SHARJAH

A CIP catalogue record for this title is available from the British Library.

ISBN 9781398420755 (Paperback)
ISBN 9781398420779 (ePub e-book)
ISBN 9781398420762 (Audiobook)

www.austinmacauley.com

First Published 2022
Austin Macauley Publishers Ltd®
1 Canada Square
Canary Wharf
London
E14 5AA

## Thanks

Working together with my co-authors, Ellen Findlay and Mike Smith, has greatly enriched this book. Ellen, with her 75 letters to her supporters at home, gave me the framework and she added many stories. Mike has given detailed insight into the 50 camps where he was involved and has painted portraits of colleagues and patients. I am grateful for their hard work, helping me with writing, editing and illustrating the book with photographs. Also, my thanks to my wife, Beryl, for coordinating, editing and spending hours reading the evolving document to me, as my eyesight failed.

Thank you, Rosemary and Cathy Horner, Rose Dowsett and Jack Merrall, for reading and improving the manuscript, and the many friends who have provided photographs and stories, adding colour and bringing the book to life, all of whom appear in the book.

Many thanks to Aaditya Chand, from Pokhara, who generously gave permission for us to use his photographs. More of his work is accessible on Instagram.

I have greatly appreciated the patient, persevering support of Ella Thomson, Publishing Coordinator, and the team at Austin Macauley Publishers.

Cover Photo Kalikot Hospital, Nepal, by Mike Smith.

# Provincial Map of Nepal

| Province No. | Total No. of Districts | No. of House of Representative Constituencies | No. of Provincial Constituencies |
|---|---|---|---|
| 1 | 14 | 28 | 56 |
| 2 | 8 | 32 | 64 |
| 3 | 13 | 33 | 66 |
| 4 | 11 | 18 | 36 |
| 5 | 12 | 26 | 52 |
| 6 | 10 | 12 | 24 |
| 7 | 9 | 16 | 32 |
| Total | 77 | 165 | 330 |

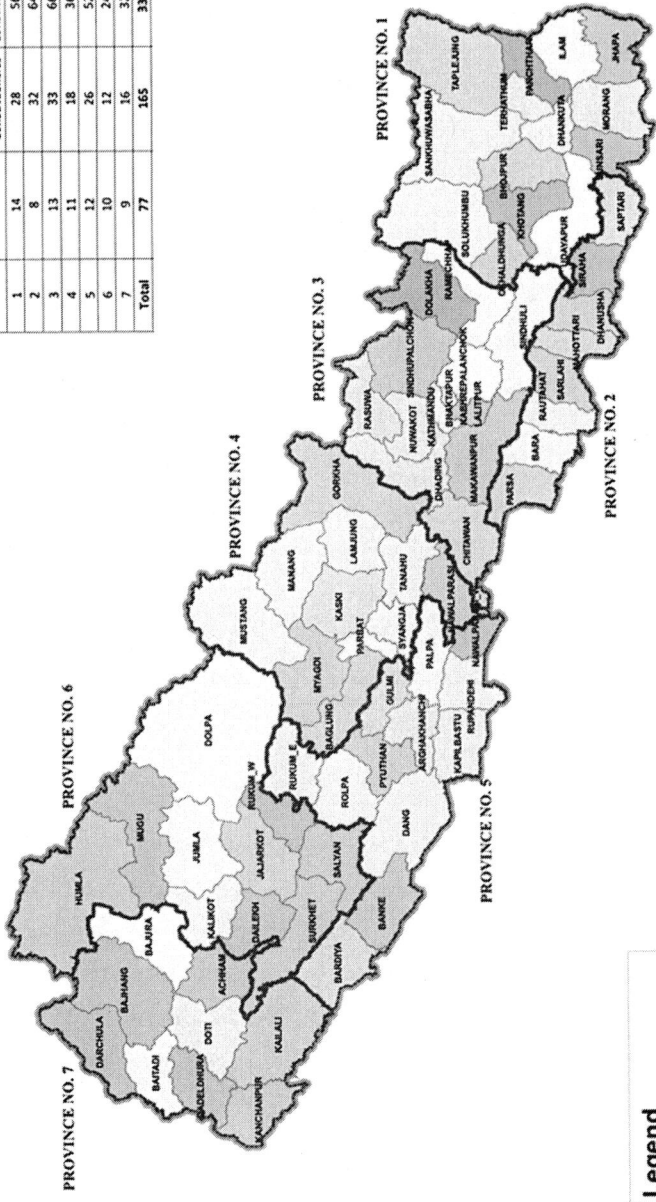

Spatial Data Source: Survey Department
Population Data Source: Population Census 2011, CBS
Government of Nepal
Prepared By: Electoral Constituency Delineation Commission (ECDC), 2074

## Legend

━━━ International Boundary
━━━ Province Boundary
──── District Boundary

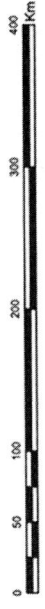

0  50  100     200     300     400
Km

PROVINCE NO. 1
PROVINCE NO. 2
PROVINCE NO. 3
PROVINCE NO. 4
PROVINCE NO. 5
PROVINCE NO. 6
PROVINCE NO. 7

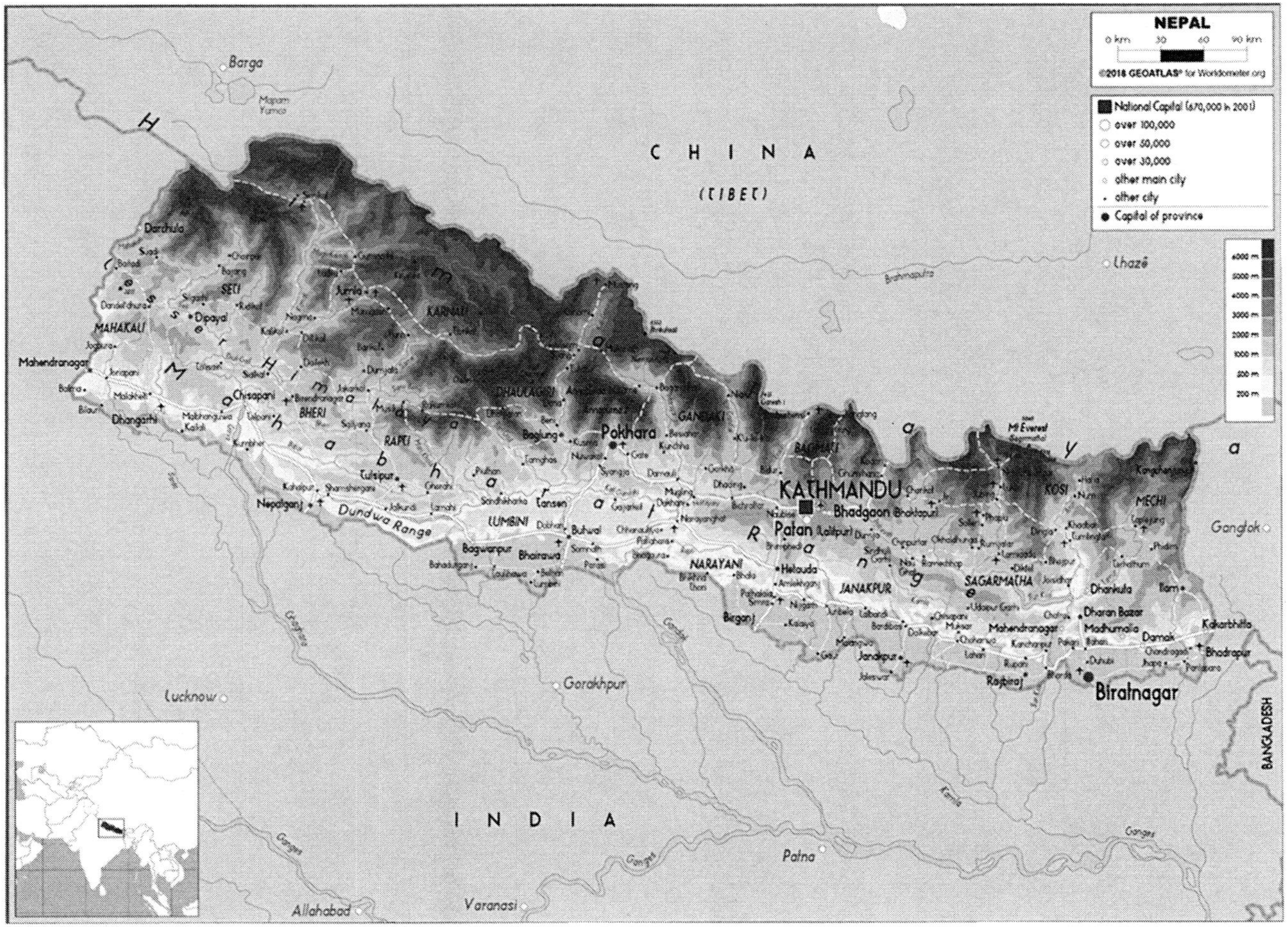

NEPAL
0 km 30 60 90 km
©2018 GEOATLAS® for Worldometer.org
National Capital (670,000 in 2001)
over 100,000
over 50,000
over 30,000
other main city
other city
Capital of province
CHINA
(TIBET)
INDIA
KATHMANDU
Bhadgaon (Bhaktapur)
Patan (Lalitpur)
Pokhara
Biratnagar
Dundwa Range
Barga
Lhazê
Gangtok
Lucknow
Gorakhpur
Allahabad
Varanasi
Patna
BANGLADESH
MAHAKALI
SETI
KARNALI
BHERI
RAPTI
DHAULAGIRI
GANDAKI
LUMBINI
BAGMATI
NARAYANI
JANAKPUR
SAGARMATHA
KOSI
MECHI
Mt Everest
Mahendranagar
Dhangarhi
Darchula
Dipayal
Chisapani
Nepalganj
Tulsipur
Tansen
Butwal
Bhairawa
Bagwanpur
Baglung
Hetauda
Birganj
Janakpur
Rajbiraj
Dharan Bazar
Dhankuta
Madhumalla
Damak
Mahendranagar
Kakarbhitta
Bhadrapur
Ilam

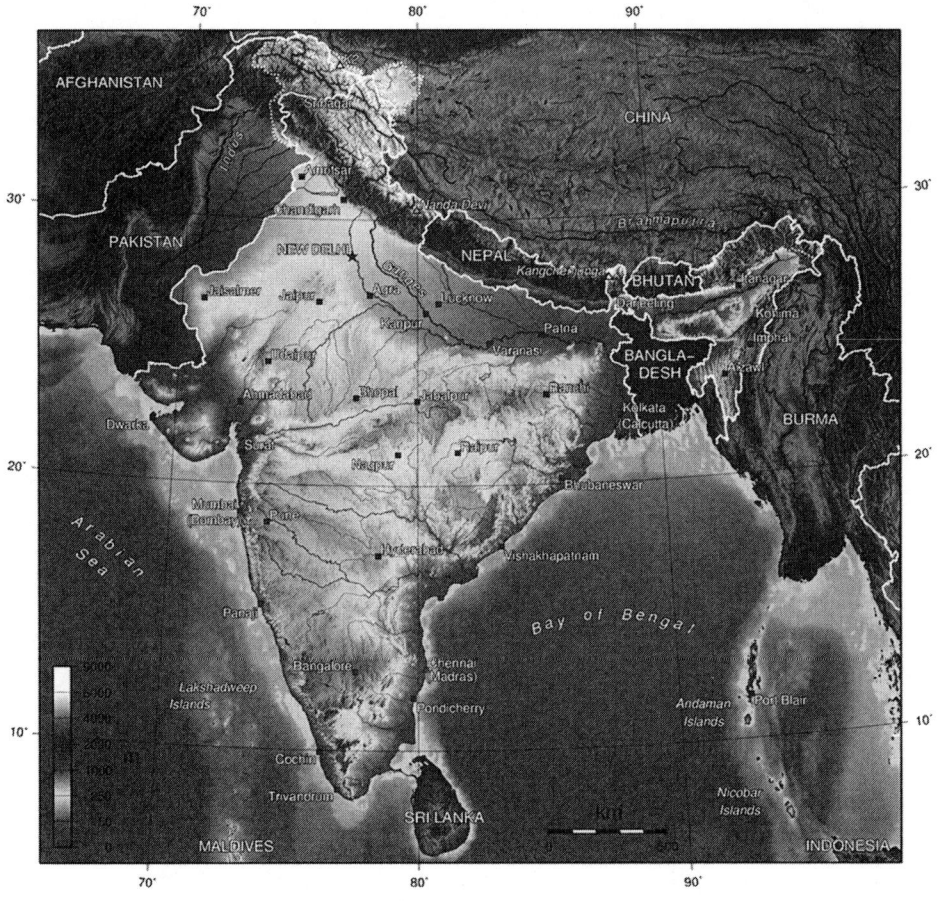

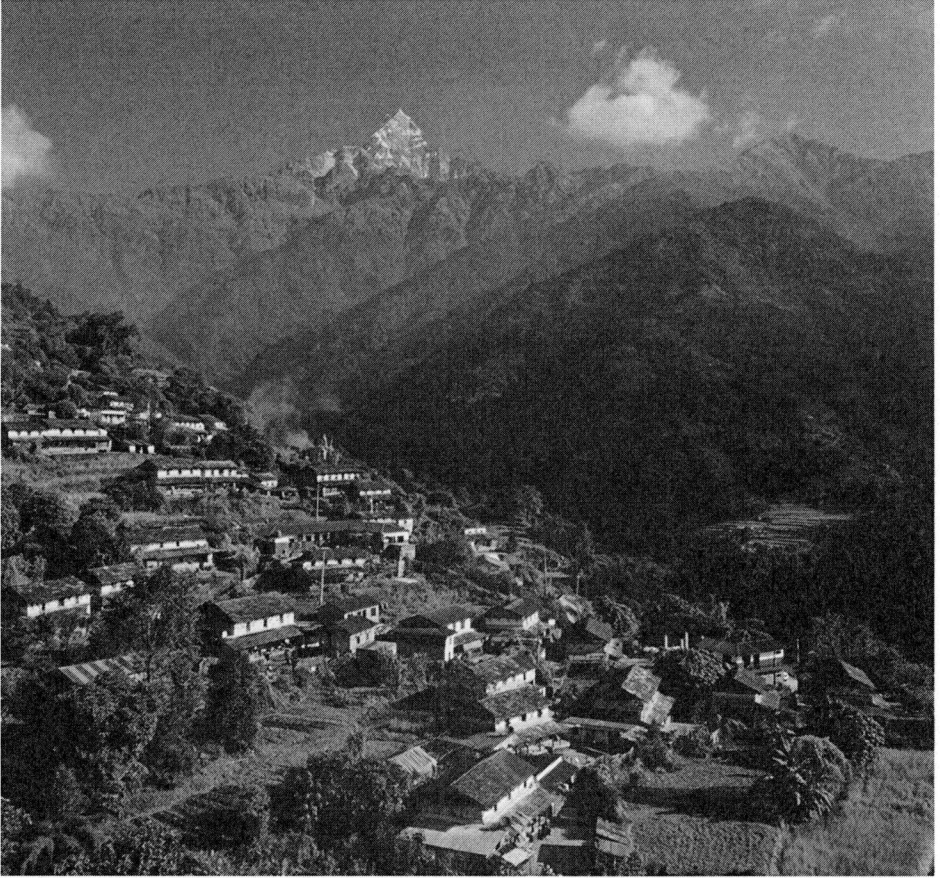

*Remote farming community on the foothills of Annapurna mountain range, Ghalel village, Kaski.*
*Photo: Aaditya Chand: instagram.com/aadi824/*

# Foreword

I was still in bed, on the beautiful Isle of Jura off the west coast of Scotland, where Beryl, my wife, and I were working as doctors, when the telephone rang. That was rarely a good sound as it usually meant work or trouble. Not so that day. I had worked for a number of years in the 1970s in the Shining and government hospitals in Pokhara, Nepal, as the anaesthetist. One of the nurses there was Ellen Findlay, with red hair, from Lanarkshire in Scotland. Here she was, on the phone, in 2001, asking if I could go to Nepal in two weeks' time to help out at an ear camp. Her anaesthetist had dropped out late on. It was to be my first experience of these remarkable medical camps.

I found flights and met my longstanding friend, Eliya, and his family, and enjoyed a couple of days with them. They took me into Kathmandu to meet up with Dr Mike Smith and his two colleagues. Next morning, we left for the airport and our flight to Nepalganj (I literally had to crawl through the narrow space between the bulge for the wings, bags, and the roof, to reach the rear seat). I had no clear idea where we were going! After an hour's flight in this 20-seater, a Land Rover trip awaited – four hours eastward on the East-West Highway, a good metalled road in the southern plains. After snacks, we turned north towards the hills. This was a dry season dirt road, with dust everywhere. There were dodgy bits with steep drops but nothing new to me. After three hours, we stopped at a wayside cafe and enjoyed a great plate of daal bhat (the local staple diet, usually consisting of a large amount of boiled rice, watery lentil daal, some boiled green vegetables and a little spicy chutney). Another hour, and at dusk we arrived. The hotel was a proper concrete building with one of the two toilets reserved for us. For the next ten days, I shared a dusty room with James, who was managing aspects of the camp. I slept well, so it must have been comfortable.

I was delighted to be back in rural Nepal. Breakfast was porridge, omelette and bread. Several other helpers were staying, and we had fun together. I think the food was easier for me than for them. At 8 am, we took the vehicle a mile to the hospital, which seemed devoid of regular staff. We had come to Arghakhanchi District centre and Sandhikharka hospital. We used the simple hospital buildings. Firstly, our operating theatre staff scrubbed the floors, walls and ceiling and moved two tables for use as operating tables. The three ear surgeons unpacked, and to my amazement, they assembled two state-of-the-art portable operating microscopes.

Whilst they were involved in that, I met my anaesthetist colleague, David Hill, a retired consultant from Cambridge. He had been on camps previously and knew what he was doing. I didn't! While we prepared the theatre, a mass of people, patients and relatives, were organised into queues for registration and assessment. Some were deaf. They had hearing tests and, if appropriate, were fitted with recycled hearing aids. Some had wax or dirty ears to clean or syringe (insects were sometimes found). The surgeons examined patients who needed surgery, dashing from place to place. All this took time, but soon a small but growing operating list was drawn up and surgery began. Patients were sent to our pharmacy counter to obtain the needed drugs.

I had never been in a situation quite like this! We brought in the first patient, and David showed me how he did the anaesthetic. He put the patient to sleep with IV Diazepam and Ketamine and then froze the ear with local anaesthetic. He showed me how to do an ear block, infiltrating the skin all-round the ear and down the ear canal. The next patient came, and I had to do the same, supervised by David. After that, I was on my own! We had two tables, two surgeons at any one time, two nurses and two anaesthetists in this none-too-big room. The surgeons would need to go to outpatients to assess and treat more patients between operations. We had breaks as and when possible, often during surgery, as we anaesthetists looked after each other's patients and the surgeons grabbed their snack whilst the anaesthetists prepared the next patient. People had brought goodies from home (cake, chocolate, biscuits, cup-a-soups in good supply)—and in the middle of the day, fresh hot beautiful samosas appeared—wonderful but often cold by the time the surgeons finished a case and could eat. The days were long and tiring, going on till dusk. Back to the basic hotel (we were using two) for a plate of rice, lentils, chutney and meat.

The surgeons were great. I got to look down the side arm of the microscope, watching them carefully remove the diseased mastoid bone behind the ear. Care was vital as the facial nerve, which makes the muscles of the face work, runs through the diseased bone, a thin cord. Seeing the nerve after extensive removal of diseased tissue, sometimes lying free in the cavity created by the surgeon, was remarkable. Years later, they took video monitors, so they could teach and demonstrate events as they went. Most major surgery took about two hours—

local anaesthetic stopped working after that. We often kept the patient sedated and pain-free with more Diazepam and Ketamine as required. I was confident using Ketamine as I had regularly used it previously in Nepal. It is a great way to give a safe anaesthetic in this environment. It maintains breathing and also blood pressure, but this can increase bleeding which can be tricky for micro-surgery where a dry field is needed to see delicate structures. Where the patient's head is partly covered, a safe clear airway is essential. When the patients awoke, they were checked to make sure that their facial muscles were working, and then they were returned to the straw-covered floor of the recovery area overnight. This went on for eight days nonstop, 10–12 hours a day. We were all tired. Good humour under pressure was vital and generally we thrived. So tiring for the surgeons. They performed 95 operations, whilst 1,500 patients were seen in the outpatient clinic. They also saw some of the women from an earlier gynaecology camp, and all were doing very well. Demand was so great that a further ear camp in Sandhikharka was arranged for the end of the year.

The return journey was, of course, long, going by road to Pokhara, where Beryl and I had lived during the 70s. I flew back to Kathmandu, a magnificent mountain flight with views of the Annapurnas, Manaslu, Ganesh Himal and others, and stayed with another Nepali friend. This was a busy day, as his theological library was to be recognised and opened by two Professors from Yeotmal in India. That was followed by a hot curry in Thamel, a colourful tourist area in central Kathmandu. He took me next morning for my flight back to UK. The airport was under tight police control, as a plane had been hijacked to Afghanistan the previous week. Progress was slow, and my atrial fibrillation chose that moment to trigger and my pulse became fast. I felt unwell, but fortunately I was travelling business class, and I soon settled again.

I was away 16 days, plus travel to and from Jura. It was a very memorable experience. Tragically, sometime after we left, the Maoist insurgents raided the town and killed 22 policemen there. However, I had been unaware of any Maoist activity throughout my visit, and they never threatened Ellen or her team.

# Introduction

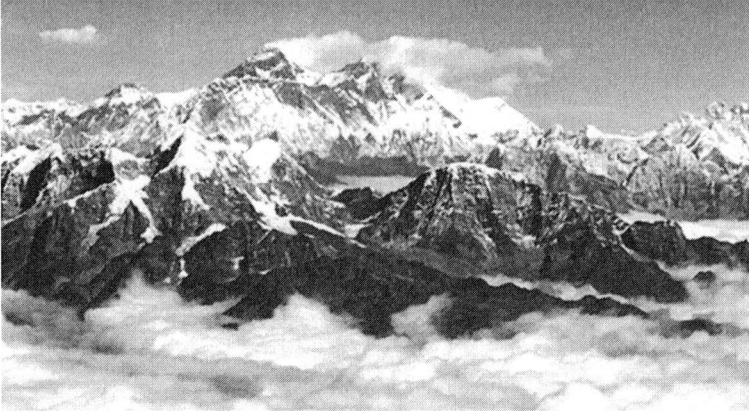

*Mount Everest in eastern Nepal.*

Nepal is an extraordinarily beautiful land, like no other on earth. It is also desperately needy. The dramatic beauty of its mountains hides the enormous poverty and disease of the millions, perhaps 15 million tribal people, scattered through the less accessible deep valleys and steep hillsides. It is the bringing of help to these people which is the story of this book.

In season, it is crowded with tourists. Flights are all full. Tourists come to see the old culture: Kathmandu, Bhaktapur and Patan, three cities in the Kathmandu valley, full of temples and Hindu shrines. Many go trekking, particularly in the Annapurna region west of Kathmandu, or north into Langtang. The Chitwan wildlife park in the Terai, bordering India, is a 4–5-hour road journey from the capital. The park shelters rare rhinos, has an elephant reserve, boat rides past sleepy crocodiles, beautiful birds and the elusive tiger. The truly adventurous fly into the terrifying airstrip at Lukla, in the Everest area, where high-level trekking and climbing is available with support from Sherpas.

Nepal is 500 miles long and up to 100 miles wide. The mountains form the northern border with the Tibetan region of China. The southern fertile strip is flat, part of the Ganges plain. Then the foothills and the mid-hills (up to 12,000 ft) rise steeply towards the snow-covered Himalayas. After climbing Everest for the first time in 1953 with Sherpa Tenzing Norgay, Sir Edmund Hillary, in gratitude to the local Sherpas, established and equipped a hospital in that high region, in Namche Bazaar. He staffed it with New Zealand doctors and nurses. Sadly, at that time, it was almost the only place in the mountains of Nepal where good medical care was available.

After 1951, the government became increasingly aware of the needs but had no resources. The first aeroplane to land in Kathmandu brought the Indian Ambassador in 1949. The first road into the capital was built in 1955; before that, there was an aerial ropeway from the plains, over the foothills, for goods. A few cars were dismantled and carried by porters over the passes into the Kathmandu valley, where they were reassembled. No other road was built until 1971, when the road from Kathmandu to Pokhara was built by the Chinese. The needs of the remote mountain communities were effectively ignored. Determination to shut out British colonialism had resulted in Nepal remaining mediaeval in many respects. Prior to the 1950s there was almost no government healthcare outside the capital.

Although Nepal was closed to foreigners, Nepalis were free to come and go across the border into India, where small mission groups, waiting hopefully for Nepal to open, offered them medical help. Through an extraordinary series of events and contacts, one of these groups was allowed to enter Nepal in 1952 and to build a hospital. They later became known as the International Nepal Fellowship (INF). A second group, the United Mission to Nepal, gained access in 1954.

In the early 1990s, a surgeon, Dr Mike Smith, and Ellen Findlay, were working with the INF in the Nepali Government's Western Regional Hospital (WRH), in Pokhara. They saw the possibility of taking targeted specialist medical care to remote parts of the country. They knew that many poor people, often subsistence farmers, could not access medical care. The government had begun to build health posts and district hospitals, but staff did not want to stay in these desperately poor, cold and isolated places and progress was slow. Over the next 25 years, 130 INF medical camps took place, generally lasting 7–10 days; the great majority were for the poorest people in the most remote areas. Many were for people with ear disease, some for women's health. Dental and surgical camps were also held and some plastic surgical camps to deal with cleft palates and burn contractures.

# Chapter 1

## Nepal

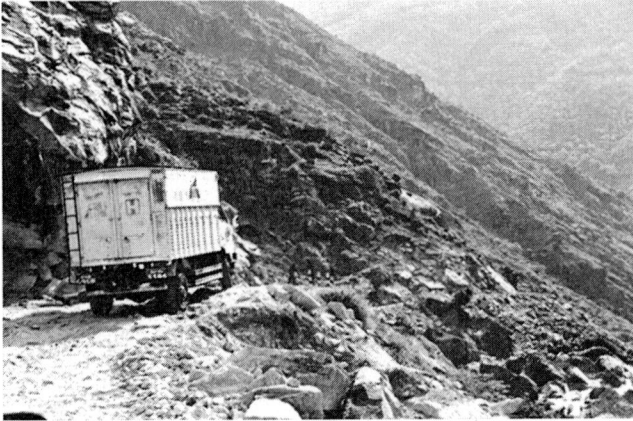

*A medical camps vehicle tackles a road in western Nepal.*

To understand the difficulty posed by medical camps in the mountains of Nepal, we need to have some grasp of the history, geography and politics of this small landlocked nation of 30 million people. Until the 18th century, Nepal was divided into a disparate group of small feudal kingdoms. Prithvi Narayan Shah, from his base in Gorkha, in central Nepal, conquered them all, finishing in the Kathmandu valley with its three kingdoms in 1765.

In 1814, a mighty battle took place against the British at Sunauli in Western Nepal, now the Mussoorie area of India. The British won, gaining territory and also a great respect for these fierce fighters. They were invited to join the British army and became known as the Gurkha regiments. They played a big part in suppressing the Indian Mutiny of 1857.

Gradually, the Shah dynasty became corrupt and weakened and was defeated in an internal coup by Jung Bahadur Rana, whose family became hereditary Prime Ministers for 104 years, gaining great wealth at the expense of their countrymen. During these years, India was developing rapidly. Railways, roads and industrial centres were constructed. Nepal, in its isolation, was totally untouched by all this.

By the 1930s, concern for Nepal was stirring. Mission groups in India were becoming aware of Nepal's need. A series of medical clinics and hospitals were built along the Indian side of the border, caring for Nepali people. Small schools were started.

Suddenly, in 1951, the puppet king, Tribhuvan, escaped his house arrest and appealed to India for help. Rapid change ensued. There were skirmishes, swinging khukris and bloodshed, but it soon settled. A year later, the group waiting on the border at Nautanwa was given permission to open a hospital in the Pokhara valley, in the centre of Nepal. Dr Lily O'Hanlon had been assembling a team, and following an eight-day walk, six women with a small team of Nepalis soon established basic medical services. This was followed by what became known as The Shining Hospital, set up in a series of aluminium Nissen huts, flown up from Calcutta. For nearly 30 years, this hospital and its sister hospital for leprosy-affected people, Green Pastures Hospital (GPH), provided the medical care for people from a very large area in central and western Nepal.

By the end of the 1970s, the Nepali government was developing healthcare, and a new joint government/mission hospital was built in Pokhara, expanding, with aid money, to 200 beds (Western Regional Hospital, WRH).

Modern Nepal finds itself sandwiched between and dependent on the two most populated countries on Earth: India and China. It attempts to be politically neutral as a buffer state. Nepalis often feel that India causes hardship in Nepal, creating fuel shortages or restricting free movement of goods from its designated port, Calcutta (Kolkata), generally warning Nepal to stay in line. Both India and China provide aid packages such as road and infrastructure development, which may have strings attached. During the last 50 years, Nepal has moved politically from an absolute monarchy, through attempts at a parliamentary democracy, back to absolute monarchy, civil war, and, finally, becoming a parliamentary democratic republic.

# Chapter 2

## Beginnings of Medical Camps

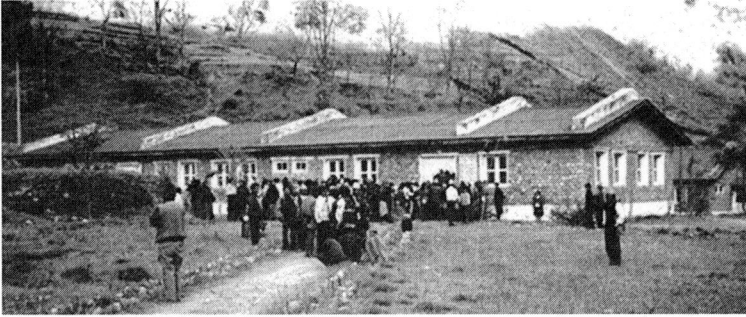

*A crowd gathers on the first day of the first ear camp, at Beni district hospital.*

Ellen Findlay was born and brought up in Wishaw in Scotland, 15 miles from Glasgow, one of five children. Educated in the excellent Scottish system, after leaving school, she trained in shorthand, typing and office skills, working for an electrical contractor. These proved useful skills later. Someone challenged her about training as a nurse. After some thought, she applied to Glasgow Royal Infirmary, training in nursing, followed by midwifery. By this time, she was planning to work in a mission, somewhere yet to be determined, in Europe.

The next step was to apply for further training in Redcliffe Missionary College in London. Her first interview, in Edinburgh, was with Isabel Graham, at that time secretary to the small mission in Nepal which became INF. At college, her Principal and vice-Principal both thought she was heading for Nepal. Ellen disabused them. It was Europe! A series of incidents challenged her plans, not least a chance conversation in a railway carriage in Carlisle, making Ellen realise that it was to be Nepal. So back to Miss Graham!

Ellen arrived in 1970, after a long journey by land and sea, to work as a nurse in the Shining Hospital in Pokhara and quickly became skilled in new ways of working. She spent most of her first year learning the language, a skill needed in the day to day work in this little 50-bed hospital and vital, years later, for running medical camps. The Shining Hospital met but a drop in the vast ocean of need, but it was a small team working to as high a level as possible in very basic conditions. That too prepared Ellen for the far more remote situations and lack of facilities she would face in the hills. Mornings were spent battling through outpatients, assisting the two or three doctors, treating less serious injuries, pulling teeth, incising abscesses, setting fractures and plastering, with no X-ray backup. The people had little concept of Western medicine, many having previously used witchdoctors and traditional village remedies.

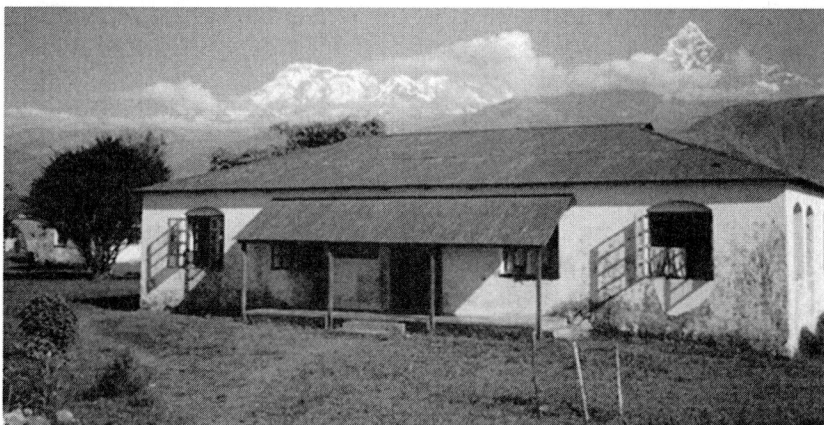

*The out-patient building at Shining Hospital in Pokhara (1980).*

Gastroenteritis and tuberculosis were rife. Trying to explain to Tibetan refugees that they must take their TB treatment for nine months was near impossible. Expatriates were rarely able to learn Tibetan. Babies and young children having rehydration for diarrhoeal diseases lay on the grass with their mums, around the hospital. This therapy was difficult to explain to parents, why put fluid in, when the child is clearly trying to expel fluid? Children and adults, with burns from rolling into the fire or spilling boiling water or lentils over themselves, commonly needed a lengthy admission and skin grafting. At times, life could be a whirlwind.

In 1980, Ellen was moved to the mission leprosy hospital, Green Pastures, at the other end of the valley, with the most magnificent views of 100 miles of Himalayas. She met Dr Mike Smith, who was the medical officer there. Restorative surgery was performed—rebuilding noses, and transplanting tendons to give paralysed hands some function. Little did either of them guess what a transformation that hospital would undergo, thirty years later, involving both of them.

When the newly built joint mission/government hospital, the Western Regional Hospital, was established, Ellen moved there to run a ward, then to establish the Outpatient and Emergency Departments, bringing order and structure. By this stage, she had a wide experience of medical needs in Nepal. She had a firm grasp of both culture and language but was becoming increasingly frustrated by events in the hospital. Crucial Nepali staff were moved or took leave of absence.

As a student in the 70s, Mike Smith had trekked up into the Everest area, following a medical elective at Vellore hospital in South India. The trek gave him his first insight into life in rural Nepal. He qualified as a doctor in 1976, and in 1980, he came, with his wife Fiona, to work in Green Pastures leprosy hospital as the medical officer for two years. Ellen Findlay worked with him as the senior sister. Family responsibilities and illness required Mike and Fiona to return home to the UK in 1982. During the next few years, he specialised in Ear, Nose and Throat surgery (ENT), passing his higher surgical exams. He and Fiona and their two children, Luke and Lydia, returned to INF in 1990, and he was seconded to the Western Regional Hospital, at that stage jointly run by the Nepali government and INF.

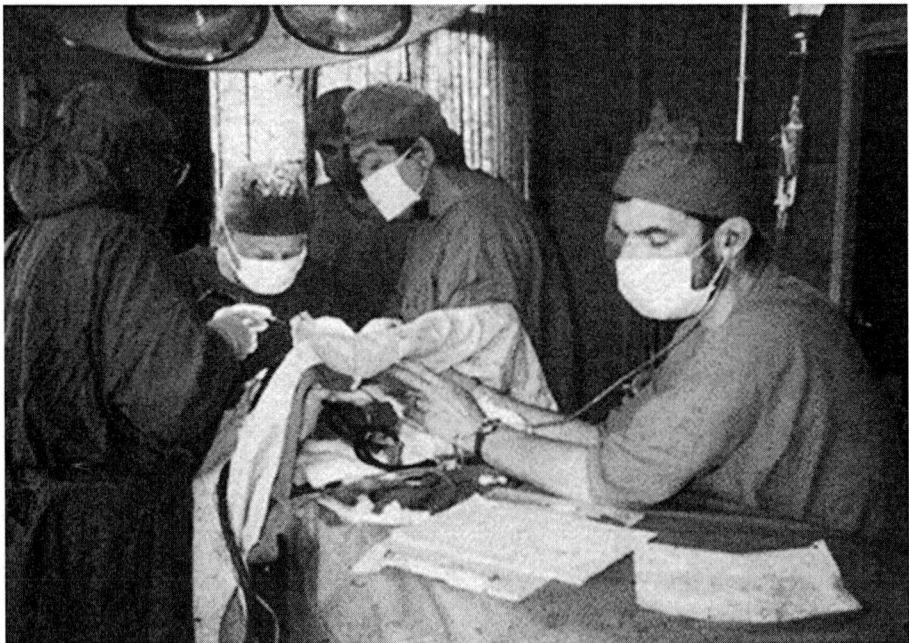

*Dr Charlie Collins anaesthetising a small child for Dr Mike Smith and Dr KB Shrestha. WRH.*

Nepal had major health problems, very poor nutrition and hygiene, contaminated water supplies and little sanitation. Patients attended the new ENT department set up by Mike in large numbers, with serious diseases such as throat cancers, broken jaws, extensive head and neck infections and tumours. In those days, before iodine supplements were added to packet salt and bread, goitres were very common. Local salt came as rock salt, with little or no iodine content, brought down on pack animals from Tibet. These mule trains made a beautiful sight, with coloured halters and plumes on their heads, and the lovely sound of the bells around their necks echoed down the road. Iodine deficiency often leads to very large thyroid goitres, even pressing on the windpipe, and needing surgery. Many others, including young children, had severe ear infections, often with potentially life-threatening complications. The hospital chiefs, however, initially saw no need for a specialist unit. "We have little ENT disease here." was the comment. While fighting his corner, Mike found himself doing much complex head and neck surgery. Again, he worked closely with Ellen. They formed part of a team of expatriate professionals working at WRH, including, among others, the general surgeon, Ian Bissett from New Zealand, who later returned to do general surgical camps, and David Shepherd, who as an anaesthetic technician, did an amazing and selfless job giving most of the general anaesthesia for all types of procedures, day and night, for some years. It was very hard to recruit a Nepali anaesthetist as it was an unpopular specialty in Nepal at that time.

By 1992, Mike and Ellen had done a survey of where patients coming to the hospital had travelled from. Roads and buses now connected Pokhara with Kathmandu, 130 miles to the east, with India, 80 miles to the south, and a new road heading west was under construction. Analysing their findings, they realised that few patients beyond these bus routes attended the hospital. There were some health posts but no other doctor-led hospital within 50 miles, and indeed much further to the undeveloped west. Mike went by bus and on foot, with a visiting medical student, to Burtibang to teach local INF community development staff a little ENT, see some patients, do a few minor operations and a small school survey for ear problems. They found there were many suffering from ear disease, often simple blockage with wax, but also infection and hearing loss.

They asked themselves the big question: what about all the millions who live in inaccessible towns and villages hidden away in the mountains? What help was there for them? The government's plans for healthcare were slowly being rolled out. Health posts were planned for village areas, staffed by a couple of nurses. Each of the 75 districts would have a 15-bed hospital staffed by a doctor and nurses.

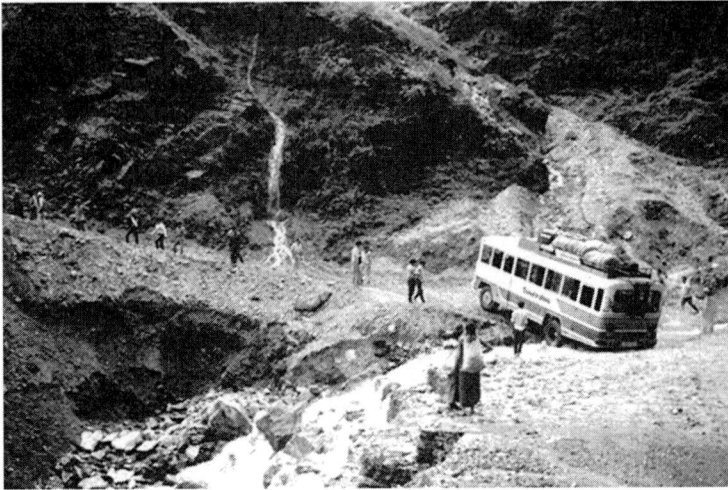

*Starting the journey to Burtibang, the bus crosses a landslip empty, as passengers get out and walk.*

The next layer consisted of 50 bed hospitals in zonal centres and four regional hospitals, better equipped, with specialists, more facilities and 200 beds, such as the WRH in Pokhara. The skeleton structure was there but not the staff or equipment and only a few drugs and vaccinations.

As Mike and Ellen considered this, the conviction grew that they wanted to reach out in a limited but effective way to these neglected communities, whilst also continuing their work in Pokhara. Ellen went to the mission leaders in Pokhara with their vision of how this could be achieved—through medical camps. The vision was for a small group to head off for a week with a balanced team, equipment and drugs to run a focused camp in one of the 15-bed hospitals or health posts. The mission listened to her, but asked: "Where will you get the staff? Where will you get the equipment? How will you get there? Where is the money coming from?" They didn't scoff at the idea but they did laugh. It seemed impossible, but not to Ellen. Nothing on this scale had ever been attempted by the mission before. Ellen prayed.

She got to work building a team. A Nepali girl, with no experience of medical matters and almost illiterate volunteered. When trained, she headed up the sterilising of equipment and gowns (CSSD). They needed someone to organise the medicines for camps. When Ellen asked the INF hospital pharmacy staff at WRH if someone would help, they all said, "no way – that work is too hard". Then a young man, newly appointed to the pharmacy, Eka Dev Devkota, said "I'll help you Didi." (Didi means older or respected sister). He was worth his weight in gold and bit by bit he took over the logistics of camps, eventually becoming the camps coordinator. These two people were God-given. Gradually, a small team was established, and they then needed to decide where to start.

The mission had worked in the past in a small clinic in Beni. Ellen knew the area. She was granted permission for her plan by officials in Beni and Pokhara. They decided to run an ear camp in Beni in March 1993. The team travelled by Land Rover for two hours and then walked for the next four hours. Beni is a small town settled on the west bank of the Kali Gandaki River, which flows from the Tibetan plateau to the north, cutting right through the Himalayas, with Annapurna to the east, Dhaulagiri to the west, heading south to join the Ganges on the Indian plains.

The equipment, including an operating microscope, was carried in large cane baskets and tin boxes balanced on their backs by porters, using traditional woven straps (namlo) across their foreheads. The local 15-bed hospital was used. Word had been sent out. Would anyone come? This was a new idea.

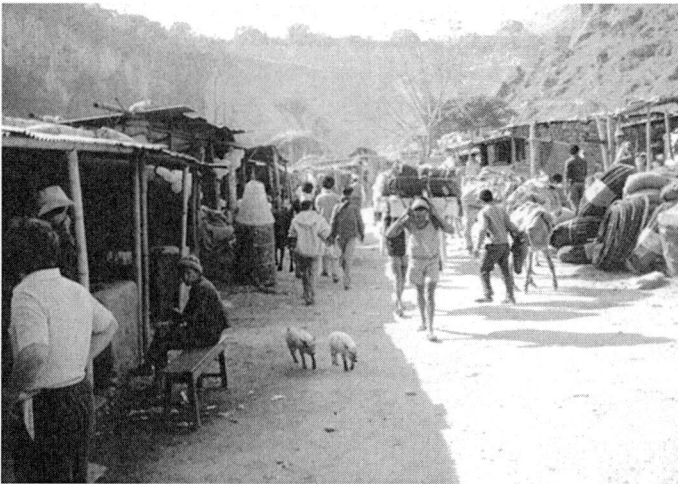

*Porters carry equipment for the first Beni ear camp.*

"We had no idea if anyone would turn up. We were amazed that first morning, as we walked up from the bazaar, to see a long line of people with ear disease. It was like that every day," recalled Mike.

The first task was to clean the rooms thoroughly, particularly the operating theatre area. They borrowed a metal maternity delivery table to use for operations. The small surgical operating microscope was clamped to an old bedside cabinet filled with rocks to counterbalance the weight. Everything was strange and big adaptations were made. One end of the table was raised on bricks to gain the correct height. Water had to be carried from an outside tap.

Day one was spent registering and organising people into lines for assessment—the Nepalis don't do queueing! Mike saw all the outpatients and decided which ones he felt he could effectively operate on. Some needed hearing aids, not yet available, and others simple ear cleaning or ear drops. Ellen held all this together, making sure the system worked. As always, in ear camps, the most serious problems were discharge of pus due to perforated eardrums and chronic mastoid bone infection. Many deaf and dumb people also came. Mike ran back and forth from outpatients to operating theatre. Patients recovering on the straw-covered floors of the otherwise unused wards were cared for by relatives. The team ate and slept in local houses and 'hotels'. At the end of the camp, they reviewed it all. Publicity had certainly got out, as over 400 attended, giving the team a glimpse of the unmet need, now proven, to spur them on to plan more camps. Mike operated on 17 people's ears and also amputated a toe crushed some days earlier by a falling rock!

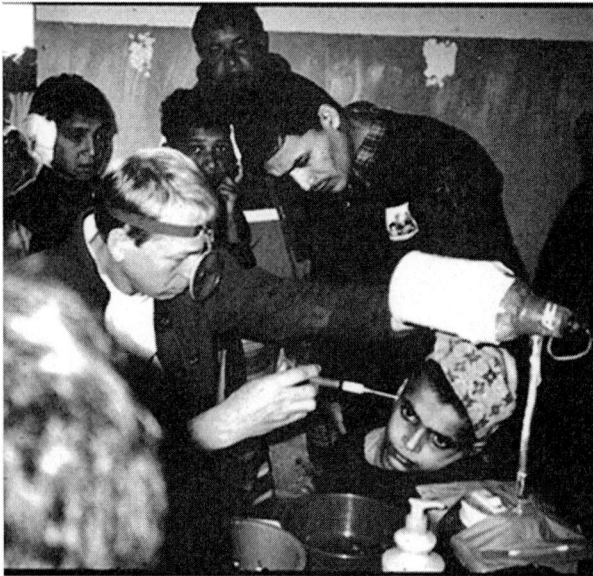

*Mike puts antibiotic cream in a boy's ear at first dressing change after surgery to repair his ear drum.*

A larger team returned in 1994, performing 32 ear operations, 11 of these being major mastoid surgeries, all under local anaesthetic. The last operation finished at 12:30 am. Later that same day after the post-op patients had been examined, a very tired team walked the four hours back to the Land Rover. Those numbers would increase significantly in days ahead. Whilst there, Ellen saw that many women had big needs, and realised that a gynaecology camp might also be possible. Ideas were taking shape.

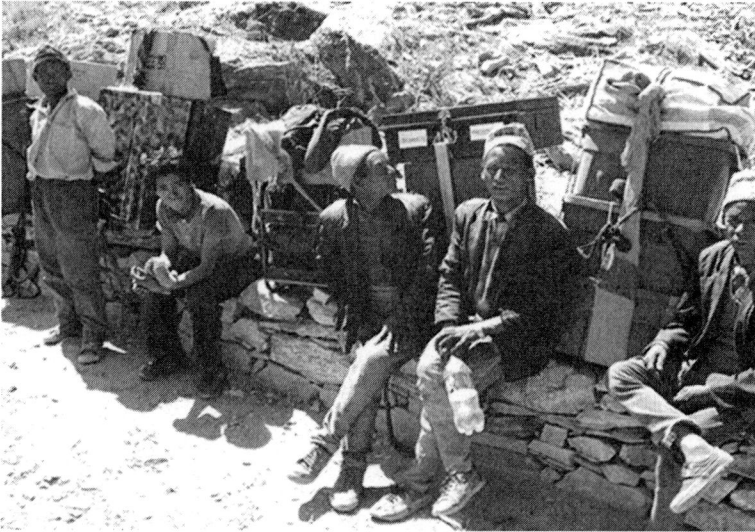

*Porters take a rest while carrying equipment from the road head, for the second ear camp in Beni.*

Ellen returned to work but was wondering if her time in WRH was finishing. Nepali staff were now trained and able to take responsibility and she felt she was no longer needed in the hospital. She was called back to GP to relieve furloughs and staff shortages. Green Pastures Hospital had been opened by INF in 1957 in the south of Pokhara. When reading her Bible one day, Ellen read "advance into the hill country; go to neighbouring people in the mountains and in the western foothills"! She immediately thought of the town of Baglung where the mission had previously worked for many years. An interested group went by Land Rover, a two-hour journey—in the past it had been a 12-hour walk! The road now went up to the hospital doors. She wrote, "It makes the town a possibility for camps, be they ear, dental or abdominal."

It was decided to do an ear camp in Baglung. "My, it was hard work," she wrote afterwards. "We were able to examine 500 patients in five days and perform 34 major operations. We stayed at the Hillview 'Tourist' hotel. It was expensive, dirty, the food was questionable, no water for washing, bed bugs and fleas. Then I saw the kitchen… suffice to say I would not eat or drink in that hotel!" Living accommodation and clean drinking water would continue to be a problem for most of the camps. On returning to Pokhara, Ellen developed renal colic, probably from not drinking enough in a climate still warm and dry at that time of year.

There followed a further ear camp, this time in the hills, directly beneath the mountains. In order to fit in with work at WRH, do as many camps as possible and try to meet the need, it was decided to try a camp during the monsoon. This might have been a mistake!

Was it very brave or was it very foolish to plan to go in the monsoon to Besisahar in Lamjung district? In the eight-month dry season, there was a motorable road but not now! The camp was scheduled from July 2–9. They went as far as possible on the Pokhara-Kathmandu road. Beyond there, trouble struck. Rivers in flood, roads turned to mud and landslips. From that point, they used a Jeep, then hired 15 porters to carry all the hospital equipment. The first camp in Beni had only needed three or four porters! A bus took them some way before landslides blocked the road again. More porters, more walking to get to the town. From the main road, their journey was 72km!

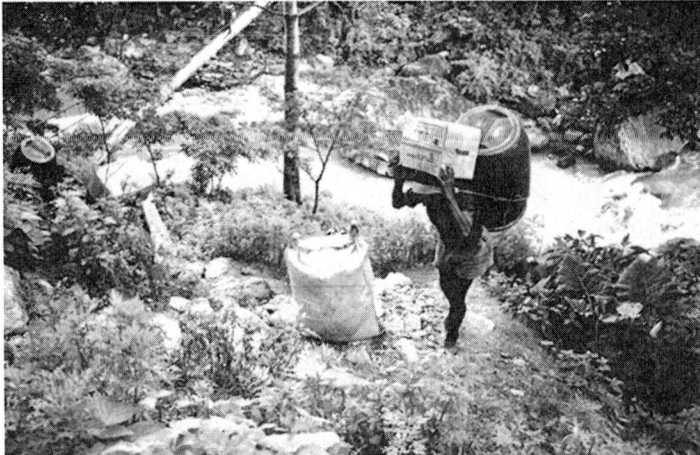

*Porter carrying equipment to Besisahar in the monsoon.*

People, seeing this caravan travelling the road, remarked, "What love to come all this way to help us." The hotel owner remarked, "Most people with degrees and Toyota Landcruisers come for the day, give their speech and return. But you have walked, stayed a week and helped us. You are the people we need." Unusually, probably because of the uncertainties brought about by the monsoon season, there were no patients waiting. But as soon as they set up, people came. Though as busy as any, it felt more relaxed. The team got on well, sharing, chatting, laughing and singing! They saw over 500 people and performed 28 operations. One of the visiting doctors, David Neale, seemed to be a particular target for bed bugs; he was covered in bites. The other doctor sharing the room, German INF doctor Reinhard Pross, who had spent many nights 'roughing it' across Nepal for the leprosy project, had no bites at all. To round it off, that morning at breakfast David had a swallow, nesting in the rafters, drop his toilet right on David's bald head. He took it well!

This camp was an important step in the evolution of camps. The team asked the questions: where, when, what sort, and how to finance them? The parent mission had said there was no extra money for the camps. "We need a pioneering spirit for this work, to take love and compassion to the people who cannot make the journey to the big hospitals. They are in areas where the health posts barely function." At this camp a girl of 12 came. She had a cholesteatoma, resulting from chronic ear infections, which had led to a brain abscess, ready to burst. Three hours of careful surgery saved her life.

Ellen and Mike returned to their work in Pokhara. The Nepali staff returned to the camps' office to prepare for the next camp.

It was decided to go south next, to Nawalparasi. Access was easy as there were decent roads for transporting people and equipment. It was important to compare areas with difficult access to this one, where patients could more easily come from further afield. This five-day camp was much busier. Mike was the only surgeon and saw over 600 patients, but that left little time for surgery and only 24 operations could be done. The earliest they finished at night was 11 pm, the latest 3 am. They were becoming exhausted. The last day was shambolic. 500 were waiting for tickets to be seen. The Nepali Medical Superintendent called the police, who had to do a short baton charge to restore order and prevent crushing! Not good, and many, sadly, could not be seen.

The momentum for doing camps was growing. Some suggested camps every two weeks, but they were not part of the camps team, who were more sanguine. There were also plenty of needy people coming directly to the Western Regional Hospital for specialist treatment. For the next camp in Taulihawa, again in the

Terai, the sixth camp in 18 months, it was decided to combine an ear camp with a dental one. The weather was excellent in the dry season, and there was a road all the way. It was arranged to hire a bus rather than use Land Rovers. The journey down took eight hours—Nepali roads are no motorways—twisting and winding around the hills, avoiding gradients where possible. The Medical Superintendent knew Ellen from working together at WRH, and he held an opening ceremony and invited Nepal TV! He also encouraged his staff to help. Accommodation left much to be desired. There was one toilet for the 17 team members and eight other people used it as well! "Getting to it was no small thing as one had to walk on unsteady bricks over a large puddle of water. Well, we think it was water!!" Fortunately, there was a good hand pump and buckets of water were used for flushing, but it still got blocked and it took some time to free the blockage. Showers were fairly public events for those bold enough to have one! It was a tap behind a low mud-brick wall overlooked by hotel rooms! This is Nepal. Visiting team members took to the lack of home comforts without complaining. Well, one did comment "I've managed all my meals with just a fork".

The team included a visiting ear surgeon, Tim Rockley from the UK, who worked with Mike, and Andrew Bottomley, a dentist. They saw 1,100 patients in six days, over 700 of them with ear problems, the remainder dental. Advertising was by a man with a megaphone cycling through the bazaar on his rickshaw. The dental team trained local health workers in safe tooth extraction with local anaesthesia. By this time, the ear team had expanded. There were theatre staff and now audiologists who also fitted donated hearing aids. These and many other volunteers became the backbone of all the camps, suffering tight schedules, long hours, culture change, strange food, Delhi belly and dodgy toilets! But no one ever complained once they saw the patients.

Having thoroughly cleaned the operating theatre, 49 ear operations were performed. This combined camp did not work quite so well because of overwhelming patient numbers. The team concluded that the people in this area were much more health conscious. Access was also easier in the plains and many came by bicycle. Because there were no local hotels, accommodation was 30 minutes away, tiring after a long day's work and not ideal in case any post-operative problems arose at night, a worry for the surgeons.

The journey home took 12 hours as the bus broke down. At least they could try to sleep whilst help came! Lessons were learned. "I questioned if it would be right to do another camp in a similar area, especially as, with good transport, patients could also travel a half day's journey into India, where there were more hospitals."

The Nepali team was gradually taking shape, developing trained staff in the right roles, each with specific areas of responsibility. The costs were being evaluated: staff wages, accommodation, transport. It was becoming a sizeable task.

December 1995 saw Ellen go on home leave for four months. That year was Ellen's 25th year in Nepal. She was grateful to those who had supported her, written and encouraged, and some had visited.

Around this time, she felt it was right to leave WRH. It took a while to hand over, particularly the pharmacy. She had a new job in the Language and Orientation department of INF where she helped newcomers to the mission to settle and begin language learning. It wasn't a job she enjoyed, but it did give her more time to plan camps.

# Chapter 3

## Onwards and Upwards

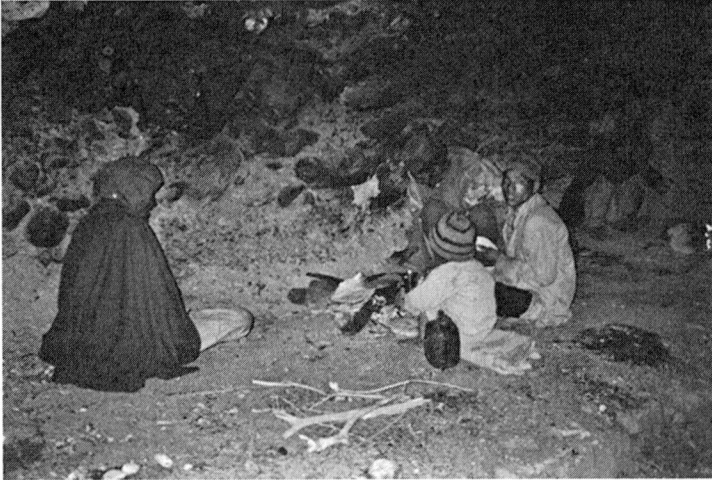

*One family waited in a cave overnight, near Jumla hospital.*

The next camp was in Jumla. This was more ambitious and far more difficult to reach, high up at 7,500 ft in the North West. It was in June, during the monsoon, but high up in Jumla, the weather is good at that time.

Some background information will be helpful to understand how medical camps, and indeed the work of INF, in this remote part of the world, came about.

Dr Lily O'Hanlon was working in Ludhiana Christian Medical Centre in Punjab, India. On New Year's Day 1933, she felt God giving her a strong sense of call to work in Nepal. Soon afterwards, she moved to the border town of Nautanwa, where she gathered a team and waited 17 years for Nepal, then tight shut to foreigners, to open its doors. That happened in 1951, and the next year, Lily and her group trekked into Pokhara and began to establish both the Shining Hospital (so called because its aluminium huts reflected the sun) and, later, Green Pastures leprosy hospital. Years later, with medical care well established, small clinics were opened two days walk to the west.

There were clearly many people with leprosy in the western part of Nepal, and in 1971, the mission leader, Dr Graham Scott Brown, set off with a porter to walk through part of that area to assess need and find centres where, with permission, INF might work. He started at the border town of Nepalganj, walked three days north to Surkhet, where the Government had begun to lay out a new town as a headquarters. He then headed north for Jumla. The shorter route, taking four days, was blocked by snow, so he took the alternative seven-day route. At times, wading thigh-deep through snow, sleeping if necessary in cowsheds as there were so few houses, he finally arrived in Jumla. At that time, there were about 100 houses, all burning pinewood, the resin-laden smoke of which turned everybody, Graham included, a dark brown. The government hospital had collapsed at one end, the other half being shored up. There was a doctor, who sometimes operated in the open with a cleaner giving the anaesthetic! An International Red Cross worker claimed that Jumla had the highest infant mortality rate in the world!

After Graham's return, the mission sought permission to join the government's national TB and Leprosy control programme. After years of waiting, permission was granted, and clinics were established in Ghorahi, Surkhet, Jumla and elsewhere. Ellen recalled that she had sat in an INF AGM, listening to Graham speak about working in the west – in places like Achham, Rolpa, Rukum, Kalikot and thinking "I'll never get there. I'm a hospital worker. Little did I know!" She led camps to all these places in later years.

For the ear camp, led by Mike and Ellen, a bus was arranged to take the party overnight (12 hours) to Nepalganj, where the driver unsuccessfully haggled for more money. Ellen, who was used to night buses, slept well! The team had chartered a plane to take them and equipment to Jumla, a really expensive journey. One of the amazing facts about the camps was that the money always came. The parent mission had made it clear at the start that there was no spare money available. Expatriate volunteers paid their own way. Other expenses were covered by donations from individuals, designated for camps.

The 20-seater plane duly arrived (never presume on that!) and, in a bumpy 45 minutes, completed the journey which had taken Graham 10 days. The weather shortly before the monsoon was "very pleasant. There were no cars, no motorbikes, no cycles… and no roads!" Ellen immediately felt sure they were in the right place. "The need was greater than we have ever come across before. The people would never be able to afford to leave the hills for treatment."

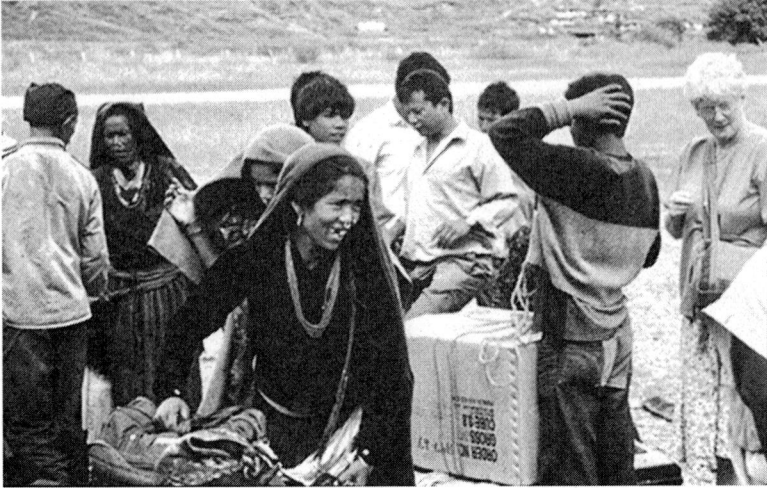

*Porters, several of whom were deaf and dumb or children, eagerly chose loads, to be paid by weight, to take from the airstrip, and carry them the couple of miles to Jumla hospital.*

She had reckoned on about 500 patients but had brought 700 registration cards. In fact, 850 people were registered but not all could be seen. Some had walked for four days. It is amazing how word spreads round the hills. One small but important piece of equipment had been forgotten—gel foam which is used to secure the eardrum grafts. Some was found, usually only enough for 20 patients, but somehow it stretched to provide for the 34 who needed it.

There was a scare, with no anaesthetist present on this camp. A boy's airway became blocked with mucus. While they were operating in dim light in the evening, Mike noticed that the blood was very dark red due to lack of oxygen. Suction apparatus had just been repaired and a laryngoscope was at hand, and Mike was able to clear the plug to save the boy, who made a full recovery. This added to the pressures. Till then, the surgeon was giving the local anaesthetic and a nurse was doing some simple monitoring. It was essential that on future camps, at least one anaesthetist should be on the team. Ellen recalls that the remaining patients for surgery knew something had happened. "We were shocked – the fear of losing a patient was always on our minds. We wanted to cancel the remaining patients for surgery, assuring them they would have their surgery the next day, but they were so desperate that they pleaded with us to go on even though it was late at night".

One day, a thin 12-year-old attended. She was unable to open her mouth after an injury or infection around one jaw joint, when she was much younger. The

34

joint had fused, and the lack of movement made the joint on the other side fix as well. She could not part her teeth or chew anything. They wondered what to do and decided to send her to Pokhara, where some form of repair might be possible. Some months later, despite the very long journey, she arrived at the WRH in Pokhara, where Mike and Ellen were based. Bruce Richard, the plastic surgeon, and Mike discussed the problem, then Bruce had an idea: "Could we reconstruct her jaw joints?" They decided to go ahead, and with anaesthetic support from Charlie Collins, they took rib grafts of bone and cartilage, drilled out the fixed joints and replaced them, wiring the grafts in place. After a few weeks, when the splints could be removed and physio done, it was a delight to see that she could open her mouth and chew. When asked what it meant to her, she replied, "At last I can bite an apple". Apples grow in Jumla and are one of the few pleasures in the otherwise very plain diet available high up in the mountains. Subsequently they operated on several similar patients with this very uncommon problem, probably caused by inadequate early treatment.

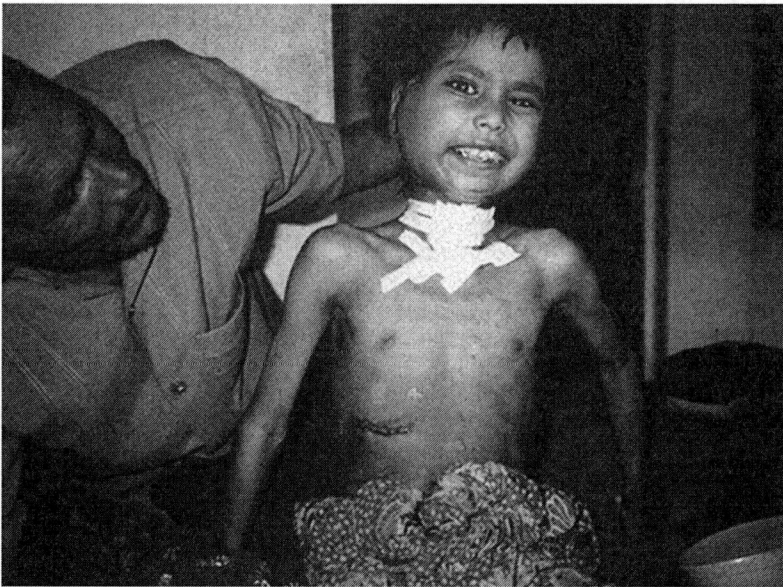

*The young girl from Jumla, with teeth still wired.*

The demand in Jumla and the surrounding area was so great that a second camp was planned for after the monsoon. Whilst there, they were asked by another organisation to run a camp further to the remote north-west of Jumla, something for another day. Surprisingly for such a remote place, Jumla had a nursing school, and the team gave talks about common ENT conditions to a large group, with a simple battery-powered slide projector, in a large open shed.

One health post worker paramedic sat with the doctors every day in out-patients and became very skilled at examining the ear, making a diagnosis and deciding on treatment. The team gave him an otoscope and some simple instruments to use when they left. Another learnt ear syringing and continued to run a small 'wax' clinic in Jumla for many years.

As promised, the ear team returned to Jumla in November, after the rains had finished. A bus was chartered to ensure all members of the team did arrive together at the airport, ready for the plane. This time, the bus took 16 hours. These long journeys, usually overnight, are the norm in Nepal. For Ellen there had again been a big challenge—the cost of the plane. She had really wanted confirmation before continuing. She received a letter that day from a lady she had never met saying her church had raised £200 for camps. She went ahead and booked. That money was not enough but more arrived after they returned.

Back in Jumla, they met up with patients who had been operated on previously, all well and happy. On this visit, the poverty was even more noticeable, many having just rags for clothes. Most were dirty because of smoke from the pine-wood fires and cooking stoves used in their homes. Wood and water were in short supply and had to be carried, by the women, so washing was not a priority! One night, as they left the hospital to walk to the simple accommodation, they found a small group huddled around an open fire in a cave under a cliff. They were waiting to bring their child for examination the next day. The cold was intense. Mike recalls washing in an outhouse with a jug of water and seeing it freeze on the ground around his feet. Many men were clothed in locally woven wool blankets that had been stitched to make jackets. Stories could be heart-rending. One man took a loan to rent warm clothes to travel to the camp. The team had to become skilled at identifying those who could pay something, and those who could not. Some patients were so dirty and their feet so smelly that plastic bags were put on their feet during surgery! Scrubbing up with antiseptic around the patient's ear often left the swab black with dirt. Life was tough.

The issue of charging patients came up. In Nepal, the norm was for patients to pay all the costs of investigation and treatment. Our practice was to charge a fee of Rs 500 (£5), to ensure attendance as planned, for surgery. It was usually refunded. This time, however, there were more than usual numbers who could not afford anything. A Poor Fund existed for these patients, and the medicines were provided free. This is another aspect of the need for recurrent funding for camps. It seemed to work.

Ellen had been thinking of the plight of the women she met, such as one woman who turned up at this camp with a large breast abscess, which was drained. They often asked her for advice. She recalled, "Women, women, women—nearly 800 of them came for examination at the first women's camp we ran in Beni." It was now October 1996. The team knew the journey well—two hours jeep, then four hours walking, porters again carrying big loads of equipment. Ellen was freer to spend time with the women, as local volunteers helped with registration and routine tasks.

Life for women in most developing countries is hard. In Nepal, many marry young, soon after their periods start, and sometimes before (which is now illegal). Almost all marriages are arranged, often planned from a very young age. In villages, girls often have little education. Their role is cooking, foraging for firewood or animal fodder, carrying water, washing clothes. Many have pregnancies every year, the most important thing being to have a son. The son could later perform the funeral rites for the father. Poor development of the pelvis, the outcome of malnutrition, results in problems, often life-threatening, at childbirth. Obstructed labour usually means a stillborn child and sometimes the mother's death as well. For mothers who survive, obstructed labour can result in vesicovaginal fistula, causing constantly leaking urine. A smelly, incontinent wife is likely to be abandoned by her husband, who would take a second wife (again this has been made illegal, but to some extent continues). Prolapse of the uterus was also common. In the Pokhara area, Dr Ruth Watson had treated many women with these socially isolating problems. The gynaecologists in this camp in Beni provided the same help to women rejected by their family and society. Now it was possible for women living further from the centres to be treated in their home area.

"Inevitably, many we saw came for human comfort. They had come for love," Ellen said. "One lady wept. She had a grown-up daughter but no son. Her husband had taken a second wife and forced her, as the first wife, to live in the cowshed."

Another depressed young girl had been married five years, but after just one month, her husband had gone to Saudi Arabia for work and had not returned. This was a common situation, caused by poverty and poorly paid work in Nepal, and it resulted in a whole industry being built up. Applications are made for work in the Gulf. If successful, the man could then get a loan for his flights. Once there, he was trapped. Home leave could be every three years or longer. Money was sent to keep the family back in Nepal, but there was a big debt to pay back at high interest rates. On the surface, it was attractive to the men but had major long-term consequences. Sometimes, because of unsafe working practices, they would be injured or die, still leaving debts for the family.

A desperate young woman with three children shared her burden. Her husband also worked in Saudi. He thought that keeping her busy with children would keep her faithful. Each time he came home, she got pregnant. Meanwhile he was visiting prostitutes whilst abroad. Sometimes the man would contract a sexually transmitted disease while working abroad or in India and return to pass this to his wife.

Ellen wrote: "A vacant-looking lady was being slowly propelled by her husband. She had felt unwell and went to the local 'medicine man', who told her she would die within two months unless she got a particular worm from the jungle. She decided to die. I talked to her about how she could be free from fear and superstition. It was a joy to see the lady's face light up. We treated her medical problems, and a very happy family set off for home."

The first of this new type of camp did not go smoothly. In some ways, it was a trial effort, with two gynaecologists from UK. They didn't find it easy; how could they? The difficulties of adjusting and coping in such a shocking situation were overwhelming for some. In the end, though it had been worthwhile, it had been a bit of a shambles! Ellen wondered if gynaecology camps would ever be possible. Then another excellent gynae surgeon, Mr Stafford Patient, and Dr Gita Gurung, a Nepali gynaecologist, came to a camp in Jumla. Gita just ploughed through the patients, one after another. "Neither of them complained about the lack of equipment." Seeing Stafford at work, his compassion for the patients, his willingness to work in limited conditions, encouraged Ellen to go ahead with gynaecology camps. "Through our contact with Stafford, surgeons and anaesthetists from Ipswich in England, David, Don and Humphrey, came to work on camps regularly for many years."

# Chapter 4

## Further Afield

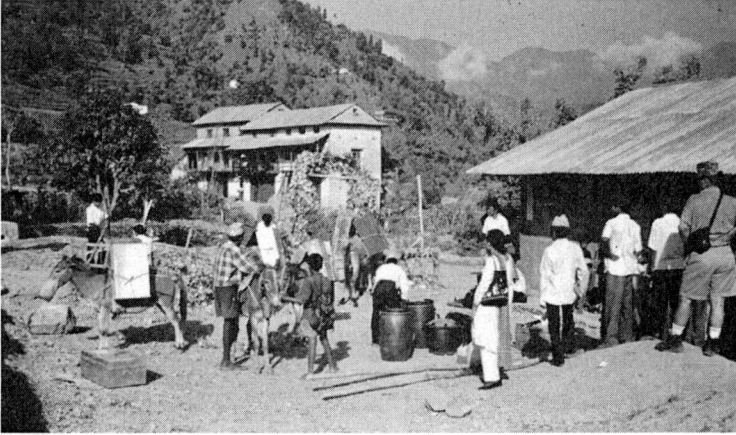

*Mules carrying medical equipment to Tribeni.*

The May/June camp in 1997, in Simikot, was the most ambitious yet. The team hadn't realised how mountainous it was up there. It is in Humla district, in the far north-west corner of Nepal, bordering Tibet. It had no roads, and the only way in was to fly. The airport, like many in Nepal, is dangerous. Surrounded by high hills and snow-clad mountains, at 9,250 feet and with a runway only 600 yards long, there was little room for error. For many years, the Canadian Twin Otter, a 20-seater, flew regular daily flights into the remote areas. Come the monsoon or storms, flying became hazardous, and flights were frequently cancelled. Most years, there is a fatal crash in Nepal. Its pilots need to be, and are, highly skilled.

As I prepared to write about Simikot, in 2018, I came across stories in the Indian press. Simikot is the nearest airport to the famous pilgrimage route for Hindus to Mount Kailash and beautiful Lake Manasarovar in Tibet. It takes about 18 days to walk round the holy mountain, one feature of which is a burial ritual where deceased bodies are laid out on the hillside for the eagles and vultures to devour, said to return the body to the earth and the soul to heaven.

The story in the paper was about 1,500 pilgrims, stuck in Simikot, on July 2. The monsoon had arrived, and flights were not possible. There was great concern that there was insufficient shelter in the steeply sloping mountainside village, with limited medical facilities and food. Eventually, the weather broke. Some fixed-wing planes came from Nepalganj, but helicopters were used for over 400 flights. And on this very day of writing, 200 more pilgrims were still stuck, though this is usually the dry season.

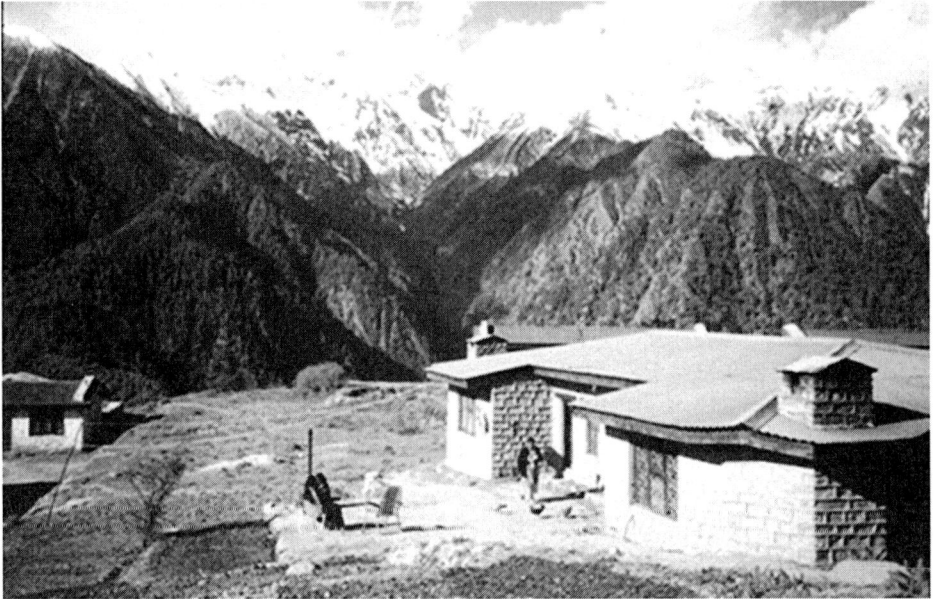

*Hospital buildings in Simikot.*

It was to this most remote district, with a fair level of naivety, that the team went, by invitation, to run an ear camp. It was difficult getting there. Nepalganj, on the Indian border, is one hour by plane or 12-15 hours by road from Kathmandu. All flights up to Simikot were full, so old Russian helicopters had to be hired, at great expense, to get the team and their 600 kgs of equipment to Simikot airstrip. From there, they hired porters to carry the load down the hill to the hospital. There were real doubts as to how many would come to this isolated place. No need to worry there. 750 patients were seen, and 62 had ear surgery. Women would sit gently spinning yak wool onto spindles whilst waiting their turn or even whilst being examined! Mike recalled his bedroom—wooden boards with a chicken living in the sink! One day a goat appeared, the next few days we ate our way through it, including the brain! Another day we found a chicken head and then its claws in the curry. Someone had donated condoms to the health centre. The children enjoyed blowing up the 'balloons' and kicking them around the airfield! Word had gone out to the health posts and by radio. People came, some from several days walk away. Fortunately, for the return journey, scheduled flights were available for personnel and baggage.

On this camp, a Nepali surgeon joined the team. It was often hard to recruit local staff, and they generally expected good pay and expenses, for which there was no budget. They seemed, perhaps understandably, reluctant to take time away from their practices to travel to remote places. After a few days, he decided the food was too bad and took a plane back to his home town. This was disappointing because there were always very experienced specialist surgeons, who wanted to interact with local professionals and share their knowledge. Over the years, more Nepali doctors did get involved in camps and became important team members.

Ellen recalled: "Our accommodation was spartan, but Mary and David Hill (a retired anaesthetist from Addenbrookes Hospital, Cambridge) were given one of the old offices to live in. I can still see David covered in a cloud of dust as he shook the carpet, no doubt it had never been brushed since the day it went on the floor! His wife Mary, ever the smart Cambridge consultant's wife, with her hair done, earrings in and lipstick applied, worked hard as a helper and never once complained."

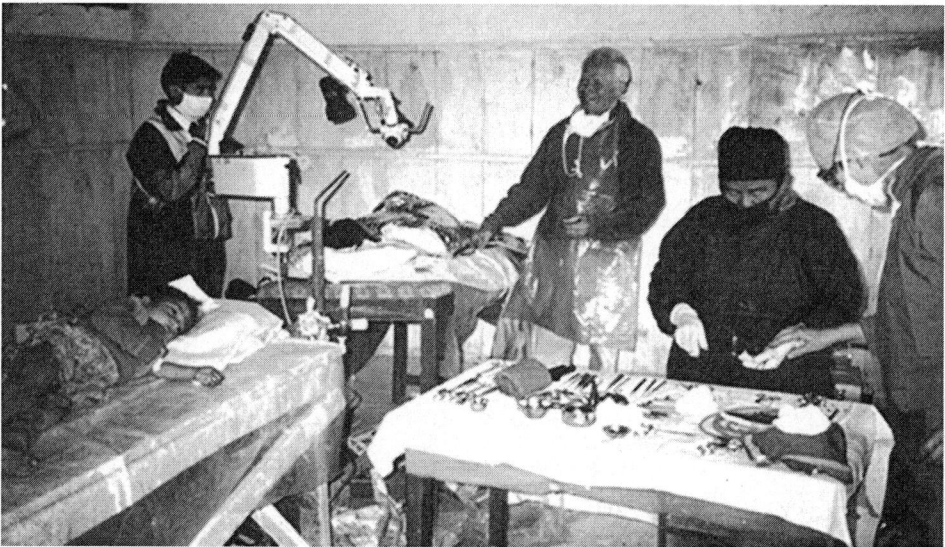

*David Hill in 'theatre' Simikot.*

A young woman was brought with a tourniquet around her forearm. Her hand had been crushed in a rock fall and was black from gangrene, obviously needing amputation. Although Mike had done some lower leg amputations whilst working at Green Pastures, this was his first time for an arm. He asked for a saw, and a very blunt one appeared from the post-mortem room! He sent out to the bazaar and a hacksaw was found. It was doused with spirit in a tray, then set on fire to sterilise it! The next drama occurred when the tourniquet was released. Toxins flooded the patient's bloodstream and she went into shock. Thankfully, the anaesthetist was able to stabilise her. With some rudimentary memories of the anatomy and a big skin flap to cover the stump, her lower arm was removed. Over the next few days she made a remarkable recovery. The ladies in the team washed her and provided fresh clothes. She became a new person! Mercifully, it was her left arm, and she was right-handed, but disability is a significant problem in a remote place, where women do much of the manual labour and men are often abroad trying to earn money.

One young boy had badly infected ears but also severe nerve deafness and limited speech. Mike decided to reconstruct the middle ear hearing mechanisms, even though there was little chance of any improvement. The team was delighted when he could hear better even through the bandages.

The Simikot camp had been full of unexpected challenges. The next camp was sponsored by the Lions Club of Kathmandu. Ellen wrote, "I should have been warned! The Nepalis said it was a three to four-hour walk. It actually took us six to seven hours! The camp was at Tribeni in Parbat district. We stopped at a local 'hotel' before the final climb to Tribeni. Mike saw a shower room without a curtain, so, being the man he was, he rigged up a shower curtain and went ahead with his shower. Alas, the owner's wife came along to demonstrate the facilities to a trekker and whisked away the curtain leaving Mike in his birthday suit. Not sure who got the biggest shock!!"

Tribeni was up in the undulating hills with small footpaths along the edges of beautiful green paddy fields. Ellen was beginning to feel the strain on her hips, but this day, she was pain free. "That climb would test anyone's joints." This camp was, again, an experiment to see how a combined camp worked. The dentists had joined the ear surgeons, including appropriately named Rodney Mountain, a head and neck cancer specialist from Dundee. The Lions club had also invited a team to do eye checks. The large support team was much needed. It was a six-day camp and uncomfortably busy. The ear side saw 1,400 patients and performed 60 operations. Rodney and the Nepali audiology technician, Surjit, saw most of the outpatients and Mike did most of the surgery. Unusually, this camp was held in a school. Mike had spoken with the Lions club and explained that he needed two operating tables constructed. Under his direction these were made of wood, but the carpenters were mystified as to why one end of each table had to be higher than the other end. This helps reduce bleeding during ear surgery, because the patient's head is elevated. We wondered what they did with these sloping tables afterwards! One young girl had a syndrome with a very short, stiff neck and an infected ear. Mike remembers kneeling on the stone floor in the evening, in the dark room, with just the operating microscope light, run by generator, to illuminate, in order to do the mastoid operation.

The dental group had over 800 patients and pulled 1,300 teeth! The weight of numbers had caused problems at an earlier ear/dental camp. There was so much equipment to carry. Eight men, in four-man relays, carried a generator, suspended from bamboo poles. Mules helped carry plastic barrels and boxes containing equipment, though these tended to get damaged as the mules banged into things. At one tea break on the trek, we lost one of the stools that surgeons sit on to operate. It is probably still in use in that tea shop! The Tribeni village leader's 12-year-old daughter spoke English and assisted our professorial dentist from Scotland as he pulled more teeth than he ever had before, filling a bucket! Each evening, the doctors took a swim in the village stream, till they saw a water snake cross their swimming hole and go into its nest on the bank!

The joint camp had clearly been well-advertised. Medical care had been available in the area for some years, and the team was trusted. That was not so in the remote areas barely reached by medical care. There were, unusually, tensions. The Lions Club insisted that everything was free and indeed they paid the cost of drugs etc. However, the usual charges to patients were very small, but they made a big difference to the tight camp budget. Years later, the government declared that all medical camps must be free. This did not seem a good idea, as people value that to which they have contributed, and it also helped to preserve their self-respect. Nevertheless, we had to abide by this rule, and thankfully, more donors came on board to fill the gap. Having finished this very busy camp and returned to Pokhara, Ellen commented, "It was good to come back home again, have a nice meal, wash, and sleep in my own bed."

There followed more ear camps in Ghorahi, with Gerald Brookes, a senior consultant from London, and Diego Santana a trainee ENT surgeon (who later became senior in international organisations promoting primary ear care for developing countries). Then Bandipur, now a world heritage site for its traditional Newari architecture (with Wayne Butt from New Zealand), and next Sandhikharka with Gerald again in 1996-97. A notable patient in Bandipur was a young girl who had fallen from a tree, probably while cutting leaves for fodder for the family buffalo or goats. She had a wound between her eye and nose. When explored, two large pieces of wood were found deep in the orbit. Amazingly she had not damaged her vision. Left untreated this wound would undoubtedly have been fatal.

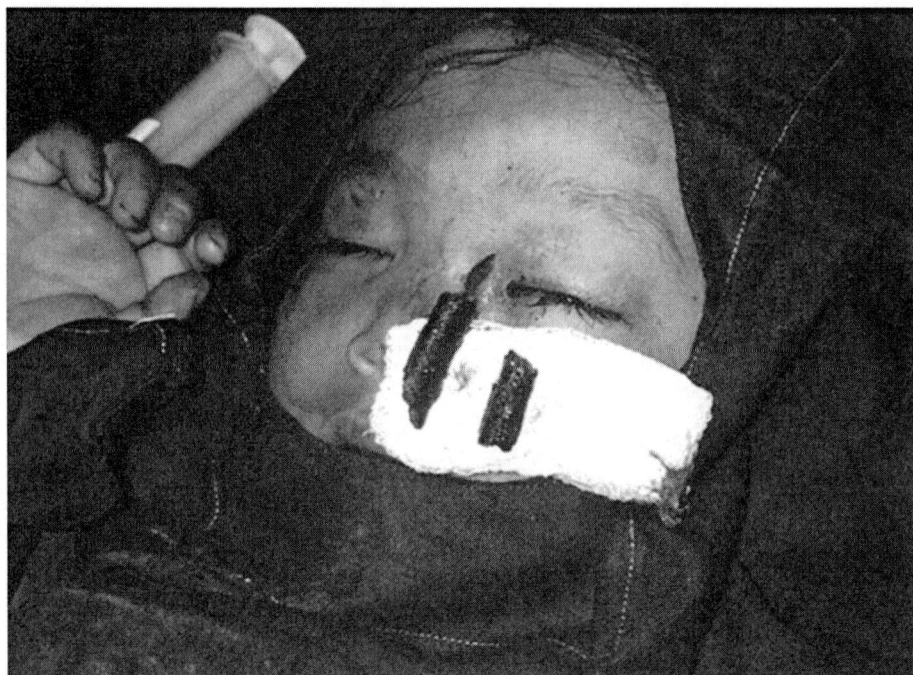

*The pieces of wood removed from beside her eye.*

The first camp of 1998 was in Surkhet, where INF had a long-standing public health work. As usual, where trust had been built, the camp was busy. 900 patients attended with a range of ear problems, from the simple to the major. The most worrying was chronic ear infection, eating into the mastoid bone and sometimes into the brain. Lack of early diagnosis and treatment was a major reason for these serious conditions. Antibiotic ear drops and oral medicines were now becoming available, as local pharmacies opened in towns, but often there was no doctor, and antibiotics were improperly used, resulting in inadequate treatment and even resistance to the antibiotic.

The team travelled to Surkhet in three Land Rovers. The bus would never have made it on the dusty road with cliffs on one side and steep drops on the other. "When we arrived, the hospital was not ready for us. The staff were lethargic, and I only saw one nurse, for five minutes, on the ward." Medical staff were sometimes absent when the camps team arrived. They probably took this time, when there were visiting doctors, as holiday or an opportunity to get back to Kathmandu and seek a better posting. These peripheral postings were very unpopular with doctors. They felt that if they had good connections or enough money they would not be sent out of Kathmandu. They were isolated, and fearful of causing any complications, so said it was best not to offer treatment for anything serious, as they would be blamed, or even attacked by local people, if things went badly. Nevertheless, the camps seemed to encourage the local hospital staff and increase the faith of local people in their hospital. In time, the district hospitals developed, gradually having better buildings, more staff and doctors actually on site. Surkhet hospital has now grown to become a well-staffed regional hospital.

On this camp, there were three ear surgeons (Mike; John Crowther, a regular, from Glasgow, and Malcolm from Australia) but no anaesthetist. That made life more challenging. Fortunately, before returning to the UK, Dr Charlie Collins, an anaesthetist, who had lived and worked in Nepal and attended many camps, had left a list of treatments and drugs, and the surgeons had to get on with it! People kept saying, "Charlie did this, Charlie said that." In the days before they had electronic monitors, Charlie used a small piece of plastic bag taped to the tip of the patient's nose, which could be seen moving up and down as a sedated patient breathed, and the team knew it as 'Charlie's respirometer'! In spite of the difficulties, 71 operations were performed, using two tables in a tight squeeze. On this camp Mike had a high fever, probably a kidney infection, which recurred from time to time, and he had to take to his bed for a couple of days, but fortunately the team was big enough and could manage.

On most camps, there would be at least one patient whose life was quite likely to have been saved. Some would attend with a hole through the skin behind the ear, which went into the mastoid and was the end-result of many years of abscesses and discharge, resulting in extensive erosion of the mastoid bone. This

45

often exposes and inflames the dura, the covering over the brain, and is potentially fatal.

Even though advertised as ear camps, patients sometimes attended with problems such as very large tumours of the parotid salivary gland, just below the ear. Removal is challenging because damage to the nearby facial nerve could result in weakness or paralysis of half the face, with disfigurement and disability, and surgeons go to great pains to avoid it. Thankfully, many such operations were done but this complication was rarely seen. When any problems arose, the Nepali team did all they could to keep in touch with the patient and local health staff, to ensure that everything possible was done to help.

Another Surkhet camp had transport problems! It took the hired bus 18 hours to get there and 21 hours to get back, because the lights failed. No fun there! But that paled into insignificance compared with the problems that Ellen had for the next camp, trying to arrange transport again for remote Jumla. This was proving to be an uncertain time for the mission group. Official delays in renewing visas caused tension and great uncertainty for members of the mission living in Nepal. It was unclear what might happen. The Government had also introduced exit visas, requiring more paperwork. There was the background concern for Ellen that the entire expatriate team might have to leave. These visa problems were difficult to understand, however the local people always welcomed the teams and their work.

Jumla was scheduled to be a ten-day gynaecology camp in April, when the climate was pleasant. There were a couple of problems. They had no gynaecologist... and the camps project had no money! Ellen went to a colleague's 60th birthday celebration at 'The Hungry Eye', one of many eating places by the lake in Pokhara. Someone overheard their conversation and asked what kind of work they did. Ellen explained and he asked: "Can I give you $100 towards your work?" And he did! Ellen took this as a sign that more would follow, and it came in abundance! A few days later, a friend gave £2,300 and another promised $1,500. Ellen never had a fixed budget for the camps, much to the concern of the mission treasurer! She arranged them and waited for the money to come in.

In a previous century, George Muller, in his ever-expanding children's homes in Bristol in the 1860s, never asked for money but it came, even as the children sat around the empty breakfast table. A knock on the door and bread, and later milk, appeared. This way of living became common amongst early

Christian missionaries, notably James Hudson Taylor in China, who built a large mission on this principle. "Tell God your needs, not men." The INF group with whom Ellen worked had this as a principle in its early days, and Ellen lived by that principle.

"We were due to leave on the Friday, with only the drums of equipment to pack. The gynaecologist problem had been solved. Four are now coming!" Two spoke no Nepali. Then Ellen's problems arose again:

Monday…Ellen's colleague, Ruth, heard that her mother was dying in Canada. She left at once.

Tuesday…The bus owner came. "The bus has been sold."

Wednesday…Reinhard (doctor at Green Pastures) said, "Sorry. You can't have the ultrasound. The rats have chewed through the wiring."

Thursday…"The Army plane you have hired cannot fly on Saturday. They need to worship the plane—all day!"

Somehow, all these problems were overcome. At that time, there was still no road to Jumla, so the first leg of the journey was again an 18-hour bus journey to Nepalganj airport. They then had a day's delay before boarding the plane. The cost of the plane was 25p per kilo, people plus freight, cheaper than the scheduled flight. One disadvantage—no seats! Sit comfortably amongst the luggage.

"From the first day, the Jumla ladies were waiting for us. One husband was told his wife needed surgery. 'How long will she be unable to work? I need her right away, to carry wood and water.' 'Six to eight weeks,' was the reply. He refused the operation. 'Why don't you do the work yourself over that time?' 'We never do that work. It is for women.' I felt sad and angry." Women are the hard workers. Another man brought his wife, for surgery. The man declined, saying he would go to the local medicine man. A major problem was infertility. 50% of those seen came for that reason, one which could see a man take another wife in the search for a son. There was little benefit in explaining that the male Y chromosome comes from the father, not the mother!

Following this, Ellen had home leave. She felt unsettled. "What mixed feelings I have as I think about returning to a land where I have worked for 29 years. Friends of many years have had to return home to their various countries, because of visa problems, all within the last year. From that aspect, there doesn't seem much left. I cannot get into gear for returning to Nepal." Yet Nepal tugged at her heart-strings. News of troubled times filtered through. She did not know just how tough it was going to be.

The time had also come for Mike and Fiona Smith to return home, both for the children's education and to care for sick relatives. This was a hard decision, knowing that it was likely that he would be home for some years. He resigned his post at WRH, having established a service for others to develop. What was the future for ear camps, so well organised now? Other camps were being held: plastic surgery, surgical, medical, dental and gynaecological.

Earlier, on a rare visit home to England to see his mother and ill stepfather, Mike saw an advert for an ENT consultant post in Hereford. "I fell into a God-given job," he remarked. "Colleagues supported me and no one else attended for the interview!" Many wait years for these highly competitive posts. In his contract, he negotiated an annual one-month unpaid leave of absence, a month he planned to divide into two, enabling him to continue doing Spring and Autumn ear camps. He did this for the next 17 years! As time went on, he began to consider how he could better train local doctors to do what he was doing. One night he dreamt about a child calling out, "Who will help us when you leave?" and years later, this 'dream' started to become a reality.

# Chapter 5

## Terror in the Land

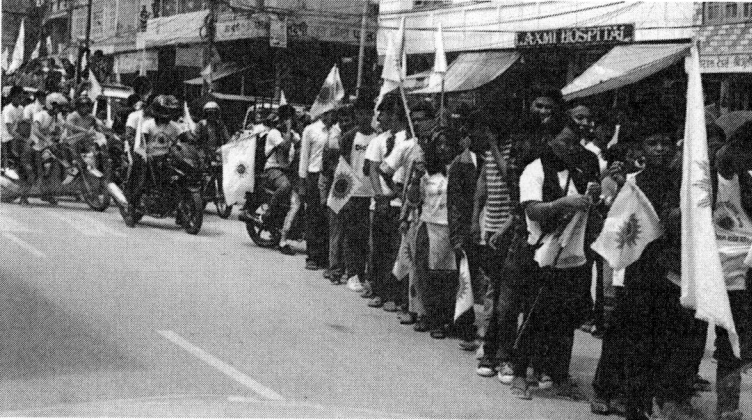

*Strikes and political rallies became common.*

Early in October 1998, Ellen returned, in the month of the rice harvest, after the monsoon. Different types of thunder clouds had begun to form.

In 1990, the king, Birendra, began to move Nepal towards democracy. Freedom came to the land, and persecution of Nepali Christians stopped. The Communist Party was formed with the aim of returning power and wealth from the urban rich to the rural poor. It began active recruitment in 1994 in the villages. Little evidence of this movement coming to the boil was seen in the capital or in major towns. In 1996, the Maoists, as they had become known under their leader, nicknamed Prachanda, ('Fierce'), began what became a ten-year civil war, causing death, destruction and emigration. They recruited young men and even children under compulsion. They began to attack police posts. The government initially did not use the army but relied on the police to restrain and control this fledgling revolution.

Men fled from their villages to work in India, or increasingly, the Gulf States. At least, they could send money back home. Tourism collapsed, and Nepal depended on that for foreign currency. Climbing mountains became off-limits. A tourist, if stopped by the rebels, would pay a hefty release fee or 'tax'.

Shopkeepers and hotel owners paid protection money. The brother of a Nepali friend refused to pay. He was hacked to pieces. There were raids, and the police and Maoists had pitched shooting battles. Buildings were bombed.

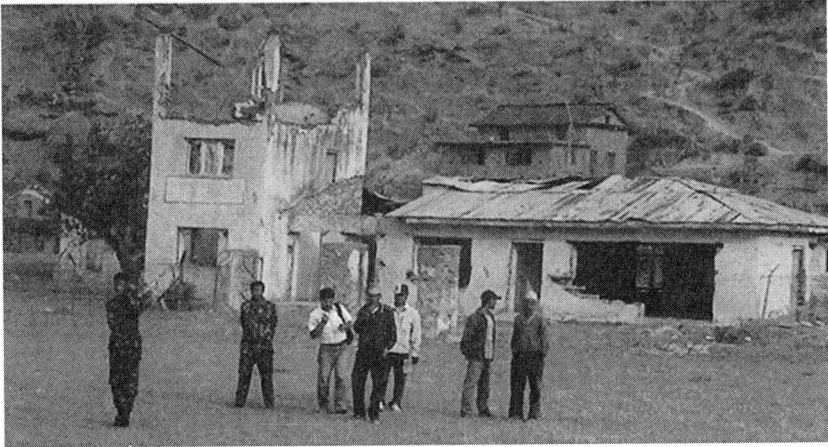

*The Bajhang airport terminal was destroyed in 2003 during the 'people's war', the airstrip was still functioning for helicopters.*

This situation grew worse from 2001, until eventually, a peace was agreed in 2006, by which time other major events had changed Nepal. It was in this environment that Ellen sought to take her team of workers into remote places. Yet neither she nor her team were ever personally endangered. The Maoists knew the value of the camps, some having had treatment themselves. How extraordinary to be able to drive and walk through the land to help the sick with little obstruction. All around were outbreaks of fighting, and by the end, 17,000 people had been killed.

"No sooner had I unpacked my cases, than I was preparing to pack again for our ear camp in Tamghas. The town of 10,000 is on a plateau at 6,000 ft, a ten-hour Land Rover journey on mainly unmetalled roads. The camp itself went well. Mike Smith was his usual self, plenty of energy and always looking for the next case! Ruth, our other doctor, plodded stoically on but looked very weary. Nevertheless, she found the camp a very positive experience. The team held together well.

"The Maoists were very active in this and similar areas. Returning after our third late night, we realised the shops were all shut. There was, we discovered, an 8 pm curfew in place! Not a soul about, only us." Stopped on the road by a small police patrol with guns and batons, the team explained they were working

50

in the hospital and the police, clearly nervous themselves, wrapped up against the cold and walking the dark streets of the bazaar, let them continue. Many police were attacked and killed during the insurgency. There were atrocities on both sides.

As always, there were many heart-breaking situations: "Why are you living in a temple?" Ellen asked one woman. "I was married at seven and my husband died when I was ten." She had no-one to care for her. Another lady said, "Please look at my husband." His foot needed amputating, but there was no money left.

The last camp of 1998 presented different problems. It was a medical camp, with no operations, in the tourist area of Chitwan Wildlife Park, full of birds and big animals. Tourists ride elephants into the jungle and sit in dugout canoes drifting past sleepy crocodiles. Meghauli is fine for tourists, but it was one of the scariest places for Ellen, far more frightening than the Maoists, though they were also around.

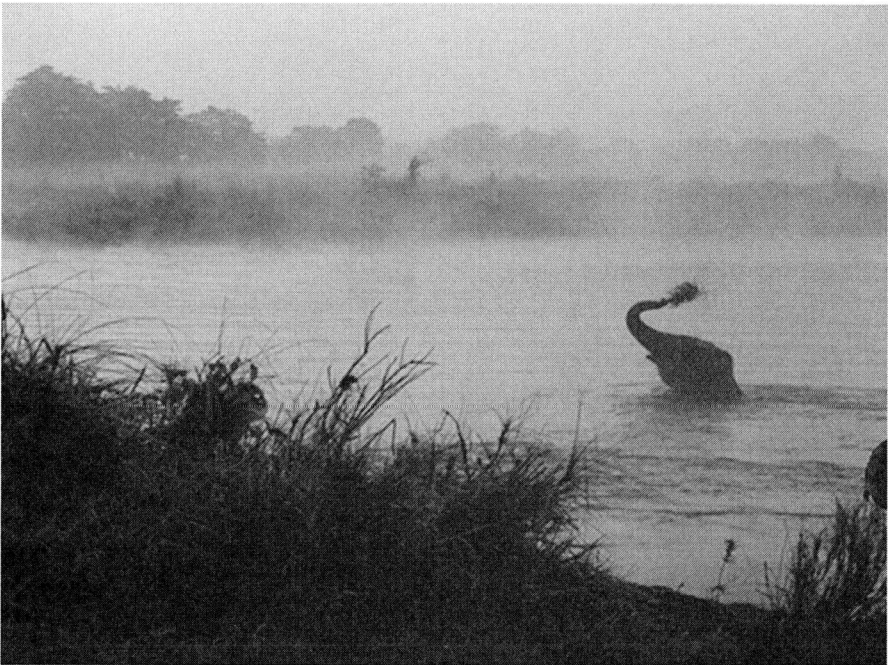

*An elephant takes a morning swim in the Chitwan national park.*

"Definitely the most dangerous camp was in the jungle at Meghauli. On our first night there, a tiger had killed a cow only ten minutes away. Another tiger had also killed six people in recent months. Then, early one morning, a rhino had attacked and killed a woman. Her husband and son came to the clinic with injuries and shock. We abandoned after-dark trips to the toilet when a rhino and baby were found in our garden."

"What do I do if a rhino charges me?" asked a tourist on a jungle walk. "Shin up a tree", was the reply! Nevertheless, 530 people attended camp. This area (in the inner Terai) had a good climate in December and plenty of places to stay in some comfort.

In 1999, two camps were held in Dailekh. This town was a long day's journey by Land Rover, much of it along the East-West highway, which had been planned as a link between Pakistan and Singapore. The Nepal section, built by several different nations, was generally a well-paved road with good bridges. INF teams frequently drove along it to the airport in Nepalganj, from where they could fly to the most remote Western hill regions. Dailekh was much further on, going from Nepalganj, into the hills, through Surkhet and up a red dust road. The dust got into everything, and there were dangerous steep drops off the side. These were dry weather roads, becoming impassable in the monsoon. In places, the road was wet and deep with thick slippery mud.

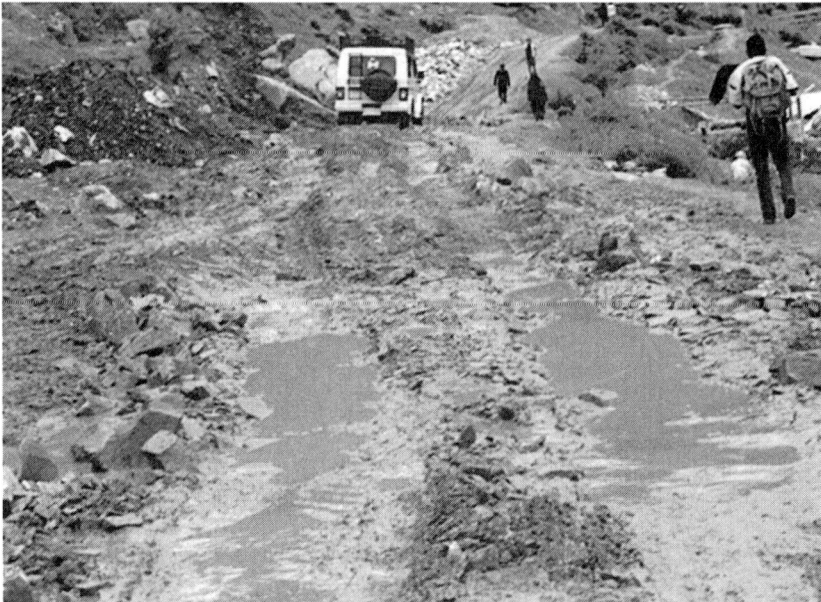

*The slippery red mud often encountered in wet weather, is also used to colour the walls of traditional village houses.*

The journey took two days each way—travel by land in the Himalayas was hard. How good when you could fly, but the cost, the size of the team, and the need to carry all the medical equipment meant this was only possible when travelling to places that had no road connection. However, during the Maoist civil war, flying was often the only option because armed rebels set up road blocks, sometimes with felled trees. Dangers such as pressure cooker bombs on the road and attacks on police stations along the route meant the police and army were often absent in entire areas because of the risk. Police posts and air strip offices were frequently destroyed or abandoned. On long journeys, if police or army were still in control, vehicles were stopped and searched several times, causing substantial delays.

Nepal's monsoon generally comes from mid-June to mid-September. Days can be dry, but through the evening, there is a steady build up, from an almost imperceptible drizzle to ten hours of torrential downpour, causing flooding and landslides. Landslides are terrifying, when the deforested slopes slip, sometimes taking away all or part of a village. Rocks, soil and remaining trees run like an avalanche, down slopes and along valleys, moving huge boulders and destroying everything in their path. Pokhara has about 200 inches of rain in the 100-day monsoon period. The temperature is 35–40° C in the day and a very humid 25–30° C at night, making sleep difficult. The mosquitoes are terrible, and leeches attach themselves to any exposed areas of trekkers' skin. Ellen did hold an early camp in Besisahar during the rains, but it was chaotic. December and January were too cold for camps above 3,000 ft. The planning of camps had to take into account so many things: altitude and temperature, feasibility of travel in that season, times for crop planting and harvesting, school exams and festival times. In the Terai, the heat could be intense and the flies even worse. When dealing with infected ears, the doctors constantly had to brush flies away from the patients' ears and their own hands. Mosquito repellent coils were lit under the tables in outpatients and the operating theatre. Ceilings and windows were often not sealed. On one occasion, a sparrow landed on the instrument table while Mike was operating! Trying to concentrate while mosquitoes bite your ankles is not something most Western surgeons have experienced!

The Dailekh ear camp, in April 1999, was at a good time. It was an effective, busy camp. The district had a population of 225,000 and was situated at about 5,000 ft. Ellen comments: "In Dailekh, the spiritual and physical needs of the district were immense. Need was everywhere, poverty was rife, but the people had a dignity. They were unwilling to say, 'I'm poor.' Few were able to pay for their medicines or operations."

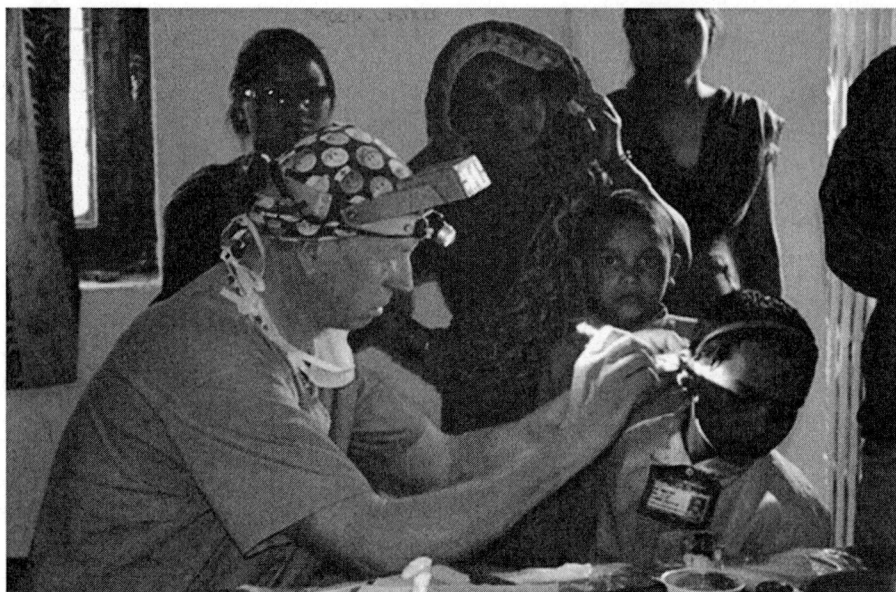

*Mike examines a boy from one of the many small deaf schools scattered around Nepal.
Most have no access to hearing aids.*

As always, there were many stories to be told: "Why didn't you come for your son's operation?" "I had to go to the bank and get cash for my wife's gold to get 500 rupees." (Nepali women, maybe as part of the wedding gift, carry 9 carat gold as earrings all-round the ear, or through their nose, as their bank). The money was returned.

Ranga had had ear discharge for 23 of his 30 years and had developed a facial palsy. "Why have you come so late?" "I had to beg and borrow the 500 rupees. I've even borrowed these clothes to come. My wife is disabled and I have to get enough wood for cooking and carry the water to last while I'm away from home." He had his surgery, free of cost. Lukas Eberle, a Swiss ENT surgeon, was a Nepali size and he offered some of his clothes. David, the anaesthetist contributed 1,000 Rupees. Ranga, as others, before and after, asked, "Why do you come such distances to help us?"

The accommodation was poor. Very little water. The toilets were filthy, and there was no wash room. Washing had to be done in the open. These marks of poor development would change. The coming of a serviceable road would make a lot of difference. The team always carried its own generator and fuel. Ear surgery using microscopes, drills, suction and other items needs reliable power.

Often, during surgery, the power would fail or dim, and a shout would go out to call someone to start the generator.

This was the first ear camp attended by Dr Lukas Eberle, who had trained at a prestigious centre in Zurich and who somehow came to know about Mike and the INF camps. He had helped at one previous ear camp with an American group in the Dominican Republic. He worked close to Lake Lucerne, and lived in a beautiful part of Switzerland. He brought much enthusiasm to the team. Lukas, an extreme extrovert, became a tremendous supporter, and through a lot of hard work he, his family, friends, community and patients raised a large proportion of the funds for future camps. But more of that later. After this first trip, Lukas came every two years and started to bring many Swiss and German volunteers with him. Sadly, Lukas has been incapacitated in recent years after suffering brain damage following a snowboarding accident. We recall his contribution and that of his friends with enormous gratitude.

An international group asked if a team of American doctors could join a medical specialty camp. They were interested in the area of Mugu but that was too difficult, so they went to Burtibang instead—in June. It was an adventure! Even getting them from Kathmandu to Pokhara was fraught—a cancelled flight and then the road blocked by an accident. It was very hot and on the verge of the monsoon. They parked the Land Rovers at the end of the motorable road and walked. Unsurprisingly, the walk was much harder than the visitors expected—Himalayan foothills in the heat of the day seem even steeper and rougher and can be killers! Already, 17 porters had been hired to take all the equipment. Ellen found a fisherman along the way and unloaded the Americans' backpacks onto him; he was grateful for a day's wage for two hours of walking. They were treated on the way for blisters, dehydration and heatstroke, and one poor man had diarrhoea. These weren't weak individuals, merely people not used to climbing hills in the midsummer midday sun. You need a lot of electrolyte-rich water.

The team did a great job and saw 800 patients in a place with no doctor. It was a general medical camp, so only a few minor operations were carried out. There were too many patients and the team members were exhausted. Getting out of Burtibang after finishing the camp was worse. The monsoon had started. Ellen felt panic rising. The vehicles were a one-day walk away, and a rumour reached her that the road was blocked. She needed all her faith at that point that they would get the four precious Land Rovers out successfully, return them to

55

the projects which had lent them and not be stranded for months. She considered helicoptering the Americans out. In the end, equipped with necessary shovel, pick, rope and crowbar, driving on slippery roads above a 300 ft drop, over small landslides, and rolling boulders off the road and over the cliff, they did get back. The American group had set off a day ahead of the main team and were instructed to wait at the roadhead and meet up there with the main party. However, worried at the rumours of landslides, they walked on, arriving in an exhausted state at the next town at the same time as the main party, who picked up the vehicles at the roadhead. Some asked to return another year!

As promised, a gynaecology camp was held in Dailekh in November, three weeks after another exhausting ear camp in Jumla. Ellen's nursing colleague, Ruth, had to leave in the middle of the Jumla camp. Her work visa ran out, and despite two attempts to renew, it was refused. Bad weather there had meant no planes into Jumla for six days. 300 people were waiting to get out on the 20-seater plane! Somehow Ruth was put on the first plane on her way out of Nepal, suddenly bringing to an end her years of working there.

The team travelled back to Pokhara, and while Mike Smith returned to his consultant post in Hereford, they cleaned, sterilised and re-packed the equipment, ready for the three day drive all the way back to Dailekh. This gynaecology camp was even better attended than the ear camp and demonstrated a vast unmet need. 907 women were seen, and 70 operations performed. Reviewing the overall situation in Dailekh, after two camps, Ellen concluded, "Dailekh has very poor, malnourished, illiterate people, with a barely functioning hospital. People were prepared to sell their livestock and land to pay for treatment. They could not even find £5 for an operation which cost us £60 at least."

The issue of costs kept coming up. Was it right to spend so much money on a camp, rather than, say, a community project or health education? A very hard choice, forced upon medical and aid workers who would love to help everybody. In fact, the only real cost was Nepali workers' pay, equipment used and, especially, transport costs. Those, like Ellen, working on a low income in Nepal, were sponsored, through INF, by friends at home. There was no major overseas sponsor for camps, although Lukas Eberle's contribution made a huge difference. Even INF in Nepal could not support it. It is quite incredible that, under these circumstances, 130 camps were carried out.

There followed ear camps in Pokhara, Baglung and Pyuthan. The last of these was the busiest to date, with nearly a thousand patients and 114 operations, with a team that for the first time included three consultant surgeons, Wayne from New Zealand, Jerry Sharp from England, and Mike.

Ellen had a Christmas break in UK, needing the rest, returning refreshed. Nepal, however, was increasingly in the hands of the Maoists. Having started in three of Nepal's 75 districts, now they were a dominant force in over 50 districts. They easily brought the country to a standstill from time to time. They would declare a national strike at short notice, and few dared to break it. Transport was paralysed. Fear increased, as did shootings, bombs, and battles with the police. Pokhara and Kathmandu were affected by strikes, but there was only a little fighting there. Into this climate, Ellen returned to plan the next camps. When not doing that, she was still part of the LOT team, helping newcomers settle in.

# Chapter 6

## Mugu

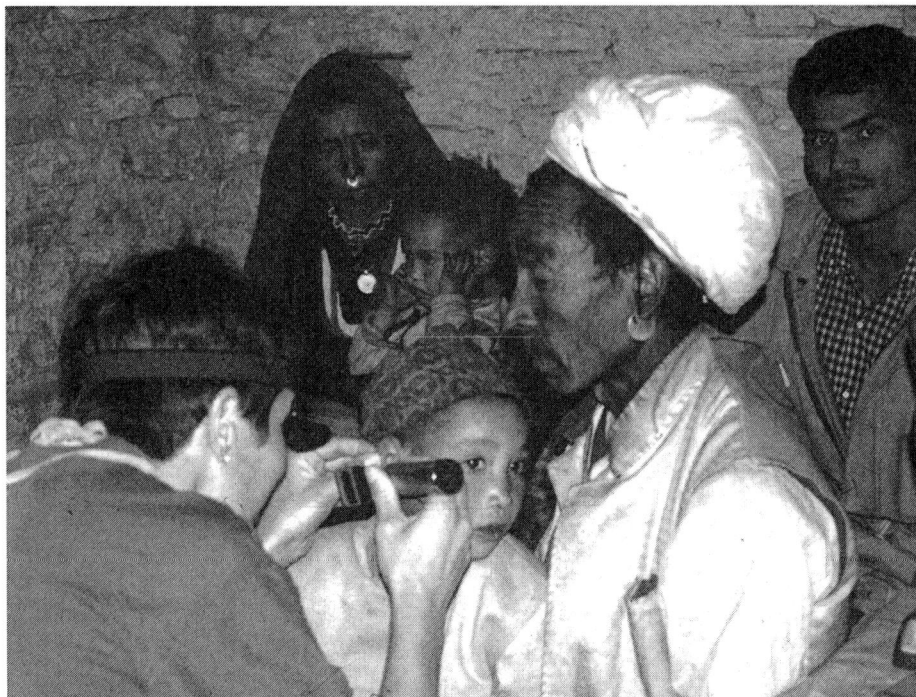

*Dr Ann Dingle at Gamghadi ear camp.*

Earlier, in 1998, Marieke, working with an INF project, asked Ellen if a camp could be held in Mugu. Ellen was cautious. The American doctors had thought they might go there. Ellen deflected them onto a difficult enough camp in Burtibang while she researched Mugu. "Mugu is one of Nepal's forgotten places. Three days walk from civilisation; no water, electricity, roads, or airstrip and limited food." It is hard to grasp just how tough everything was about Mugu. It is the largest district in Nepal but with a population of only about 55,000, scattered among many villages. It is at high altitude, with enormous hills and valleys, the sparsely populated area averaging over 9,000 ft. It borders Tibet to the north, with high snowy Himalayan peaks.

Today, village development programmes have made a significant difference, and it is now on a trekking route to Rara, Nepal's largest lake. The Red Cross thought Jumla had one of the highest under-5 mortality rates, but a two day walk west would have brought them to Mugu, where in 1999, it was thought that under-5 mortality was 60%. We can barely imagine the desperate situation for hungry or sick people in that district.

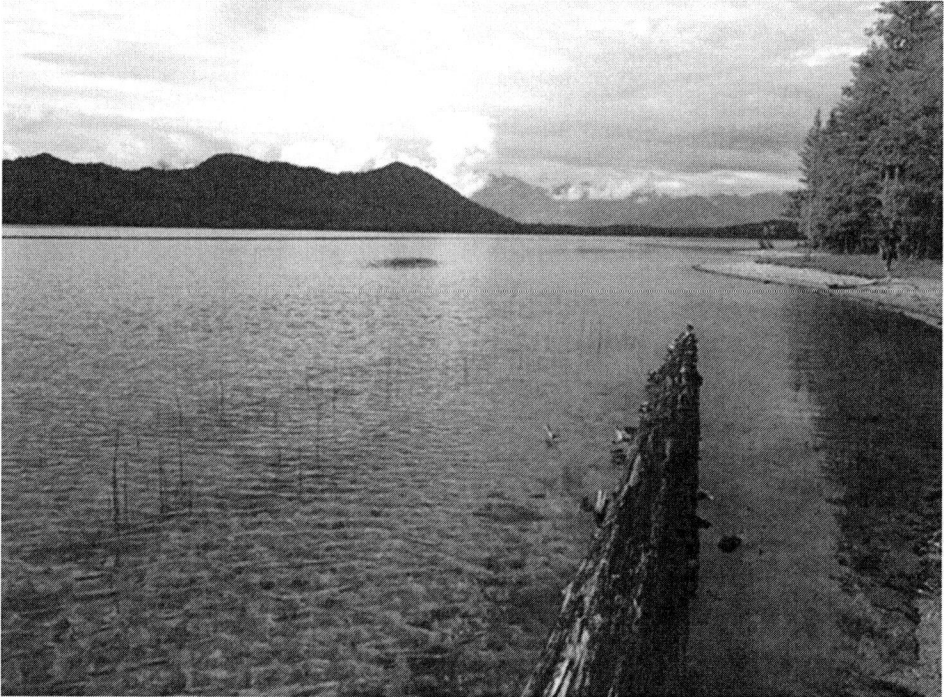

*Rara lake from the southern shore, crystal clear, with clouds obscuring the distant snowy peaks.*

Ellen thought, then planned. Marieke had said there was no money from her budget to help with the costs. This was going to be very expensive. To walk in from the roadhead took three days with porters and visiting surgeons. Lukas Eberle agreed to help fund the camp. The total team size was about 25. This camp had to be reached by helicopter. Just then, a letter arrived saying $1,000 was on its way from a supporter. That was all the confirmation Ellen needed. Camp was on.

The helicopter had to land in the school playing field high up on the ridge that forms the backbone of Gamgadhi, the district centre of Mugu. When they came to leave, there was much uncertainty about when the helicopter would come; they sat and waited till they heard the beating of the rotors, then ran down to the school. Gamgadhi is near lake Rara, famous as a remote beauty spot in Nepal. As they flew out, Mike, sitting in the doorway to the pilot's cabin, asked if he would show them the lake. The pilot said: "Do you want to get your feet wet?" He sped down across the surface, just metres above the water, Mike and Ellen who could see out of the front of the helicopter, were excited, but their team members behind, who heard nothing above the engine noise, had no idea what was happening. They could only see dimly from the crazed old side windows and were shocked as they flew close over a ridge covered in pines and down low, creating waves on the water. They thought they were going to crash and were frightened.

I am writing about the year 2000. There would be much improvement in the next 20 years. This is Ellen's description of the hospital as she found it then:

"The hospital was a shell. No cement on the walls or floor. The floor was red dust and stones. Every afternoon the wind picked up and blew the dry dust all over the operating equipment. We sealed the floor and windows with plastic sheeting. Children sat with flies all over their faces, not bothering to wipe them away, they were so used to it. No electricity (but we had our generator and fuel). No water (but we had barrels we could fill from a nearby standpipe). No local doctor, an inactive health worker, a non-functioning administration, no inpatient beds, no nursing staff, no functioning toilets, and an empty accommodation block." It is probable that staff had been allocated to the hospital, but what was the point in being there? For a city-trained doctor with no local social contacts, it was easy to see why they fled back to the cities. This was often the situation in the remote parts and pay was very poor. This was the picture of Mugu.

"Were we needed? One man summed up the medical care in Mugu. 'If we are ill and there is no doctor, we go to the Health Post in the bazaar. If they have no medicine, we go home and die.' We were needed, desperately needed. In this poor, scattered community, 960 ear patients came. Then we also had eye, chest, ante-natal patients, those with injuries, burn contractures. One man walked— think about it—four days with his infant with an imperforate anus. What could we do? We paid for him with the child to go to Pokhara. Maybe we should have come with a general medical camp first, but the ear disease occupied the time. Without surgery, one 6-year-old child would have died. The surgical team got on with their work in far from ideal conditions.

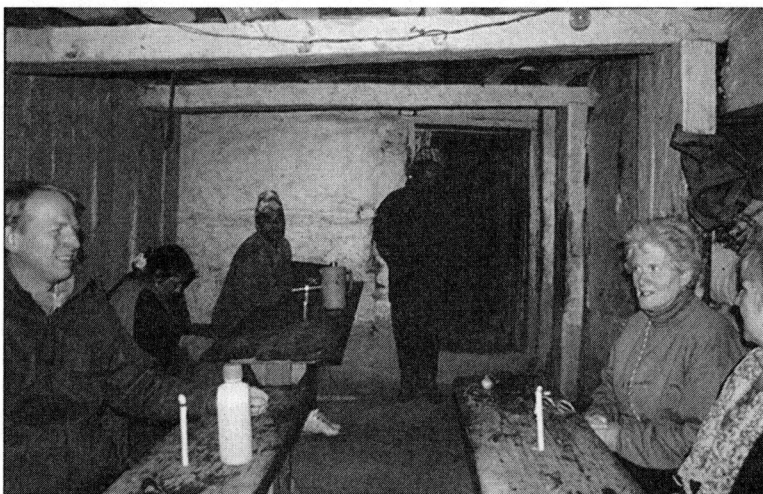

*Waiting for a candle-lit dinner at the hotel in Gamgadhi!*

"Two men walked five days, bringing their sons for ear operations. They carried their rice, cooked it by the roadside, slept in whatever shelter they could find. They had no money. We paid 'hotel' costs for them and for others. Fortunately, the Government administrator located extra rice for the hotel to feed the patients and the influx of relatives who came with them." Mugu produced enough food for only six months on these high hills. The team took bags of lentils, beans and rice with them. Their accommodation, of course was poor. Yet it went smoothly. "We did what we could for non-ear patients."

A year later, a gynaecology camp was held in Mugu. 800 women were seen and 32 operated on. Some of the people asked:

"Why do you do this for us?"

"You are earning a lot of merit." (It is assumed that 'gaining merit' is the reason people do 'good works', or because foreign governments are paying big wages).

"Nobody else bothers with us."

"I've spent 60,000 rupees (£600) to get help for my wife, but you operate for nothing and then say it is not to gain merit!"

"You are like gods to us." They could not believe that it was out of gratitude to God that we did this.

"We could get a helicopter and leave the dirt, hunger, lack of toilets, water and electricity, fruit and vegetables, an abundance of fleas and bed bugs behind us and come down to a shower, a good bed and food. The people of Mugu are constantly dirty and hungry."

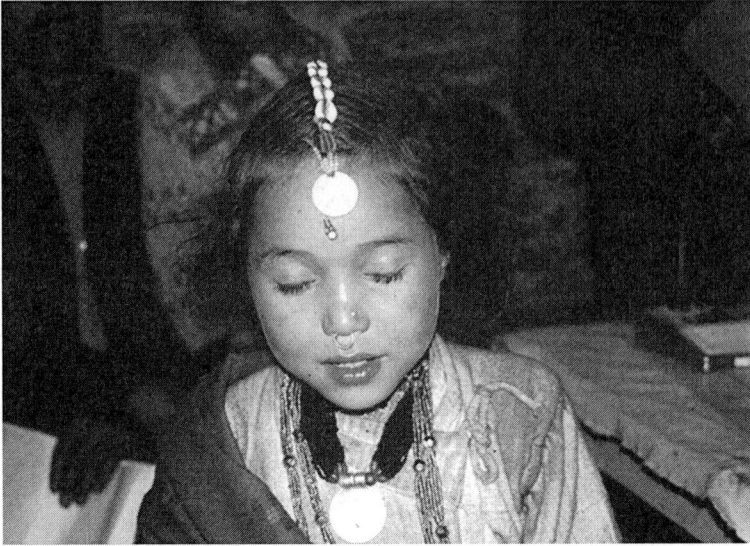

*A beautiful young girl in colourful traditional dress blinks at the camera flash. Small cowrie shells in her hair and old Indian silver rupee coins as jewellery.*

The needs of Gamgadhi and the rest of Mugu District were vast. It could seem wrong to rush in, then helicopter out, leaving such need. It did, however, demonstrate to INF and others that long-term work was urgently needed to begin a Community Development project there.

"In my seven years of camps, I have never seen such need."

The year 2000 saw just three camps. 2001 would bring nine, with all the planning, team assembling and equipping that would require. It was going to get busy. One of the gynae camps was in remote Humla, where six men carried in a woman who was screaming with pain. Ellen reported, "It was obvious she had cancer and was beyond medical care. Strong painkillers were prescribed but when we saw her the next day, she was still in pain. I was about to tell her there was nothing we could do, when I thought 'I must talk to her a little about God, who understands.' Then a remarkable thing happened; her whole countenance changed. She was at peace. She turned to her husband and said, 'You listen to what she says.' She slept without any sedation. When I went in the next morning to see her, she was gone. Her husband and son had taken her home."

# Chapter 7

## The Needy Plains

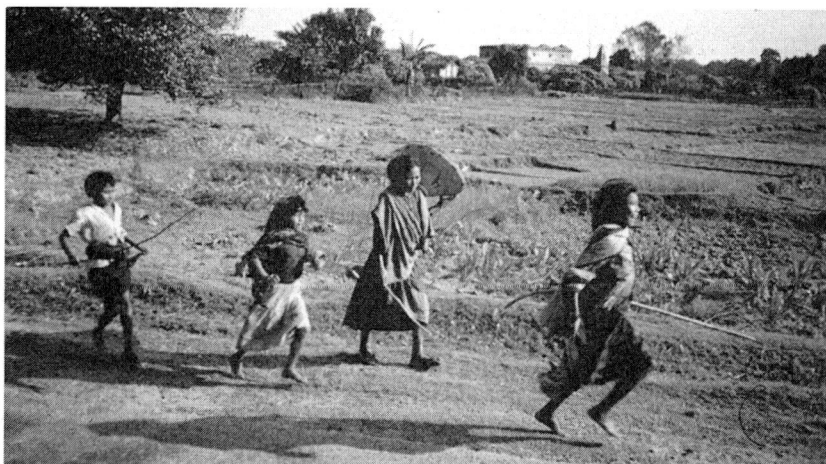

*Terai children.*

Much of the southern 10-mile-wide strip of Nepal (the Terai) is very flat, part of the Ganges Plain, just 300 ft above sea level and 1,000 miles from the sea. The second camp of 2001 was different, going to multiple villages where the Kamaiya people lived. These are some of the most unfortunate people in Nepal. They live scattered along the Terai, close to the India/Nepal border. Roads in this area are generally good, so access, for a change, was not difficult. But it gets very hot and wet, except in the four winter months.

The Kamaiyas were bonded agricultural labourers, in other words slaves, owned for generations. Families could not escape increasing debt to their owners. Their landlords might give them land to work and then take a chunk of the produce. In July 2000, the Nepali government passed a law to liberate all 200,000 of them and to give them land on which to build a house. Sadly, the money did not follow the freedom, and these people, now known as ex-Kamaiyas, were very poor. The government promised to resettle and rehabilitate them in Western Nepal but failed to do so. The ex-Kamaiyas sought peacefully to occupy public land but met resistance from the police, who baton charged them. In response, the East-West highway was blocked for a day. It was into this situation that a 14-strong team went to run a general medical camp for 13 days.

"The Ex-Kamaiyas were living in shelters made of branches, dry leaves, sometimes a piece of plastic over the roof and cardboard for walls. We only had toilets in two camps—built for us: one a shelter with corrugated iron around a tree, the other with leaf walls being eaten by the cows! Writing down what we saw will never convey the extent of the illness and poverty. Their diet was boiled rice, salt and ground chilli."

Small wonder then that the team saw many diseases resulting from malnutrition: anaemia, lethargy, weakness, skin and muscle pain from vitamin deficiency, intestinal parasites, ear and eye infections. There were general problems of hernias and hydroceles (a cyst in the scrotum, sometimes so large it hindered walking, but readily correctible with surgery). Two children had hepatitis and there was much TB and chest infections. The team moved from camp to camp; 4,300 patients were examined and treated. Their four vehicles travelled between them a total of 8,630km, with only one serious breakdown.

"A father brought his 12-month-old baby and three-year-old with severe malnutrition and chest infections. They were limp. Too weak, the parents were unable to build a shelter and just lived under a tree. After a day of food and antibiotics, transformation was beginning. We gave them extra food, clothing and money." This story was often repeated. The team gave oil, soya, rice, lentils and eggs—all items available locally if you had money. They gave out £3,500 in food, clothing and money—all money sent as gifts from home countries. It was clear that what was given would last only a few days, but it gave hope and allowed some to find work. The ongoing problem, however, was for the government to resolve.

Reviewing, Ellen reflected: "May our little give them hope for the future. I am feeling worn and weary. Since November, we have had one camp after another. After the ear camp in Mugu in November, we had a busy and cold gynaecology camp in January. We examined and treated 1,200 women and operated on 80 people. Now we have just finished seeing 4,300 patients in the Terai, and in March we go on an ear camp again, in an area where the Maoists are active." [This ear camp was the one described by the author in the Foreword]

On the evening of June 1, 2001, a truly horrific tragedy unfolded which would result, a few years later, in radical political change. The Royal Family were massacred at a monthly family party in the Palace in Kathmandu. The King and Queen, their two younger children and five other family members were gunned down, not by the Maoists but, probably, by the Crown Prince. Kathmandu can never have seen a day like that. The nine cremations were performed at the burning ghats at Pashupatinath temple. The Crown Prince died four days later, having been crowned King, whilst unconscious, in accordance with the law. The grief of the nation was deep and long.

Gyanendra, the dead king's brother, who had been abroad at the time of the shooting, was crowned. He turned away from Birendra's democratisation and took complete control to battle against the Maoists. The whole situation deteriorated, and before peace was restored in 2006, many thousands of people had been killed. It was in this atmosphere of fear, disruption and danger, that INF camps continued, virtually unhindered. Sometimes, Maoists would reiterate the assurance to our Nepali team members, "Don't worry, we will not harm you; you are doing what we want, serving the poor." They also came as patients, as did police and many other officials; the team did not discriminate in any way. On a few camps, an armed guard was assigned to the outpatient area by the local military to try and prevent any trouble.

However, it could still be nerve-wracking having the responsibility of taking foreign visitors into this situation. Some alarming sights came into view on roads, with police check-posts surrounded by sandbags and barbed wire, military police at junctions with guns and some police stations and airport buildings that had been attacked and blown up. Most main roads had check-posts and police or military personnel doing searches of vehicles, but generally they waved us on once we explained our work. Ellen was phlegmatic, most of the time.

# Chapter 8

## District Hospitals

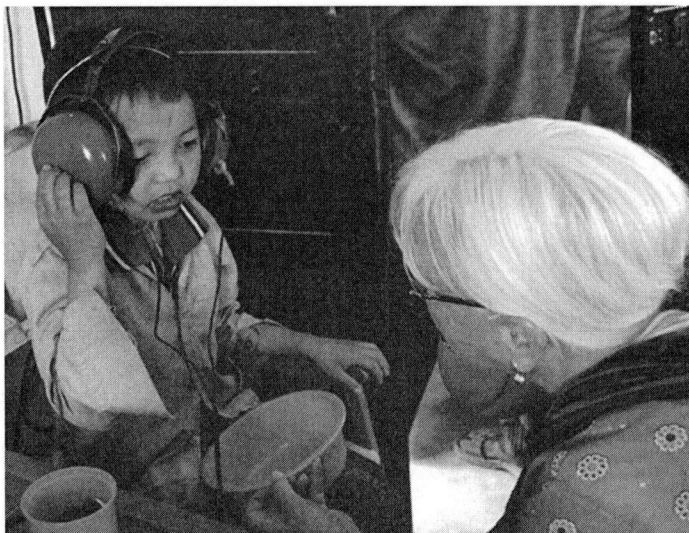

*Peggy Franks, an Australian nurse who has spent many years working in Nepal, helps reassure, and test a young boy's hearing.*

Almost every camp took place in a district hospital. These were simple affairs, consisting of several single-story buildings around a compound. They were mostly built from rocks and cement and had an out-patient clinic area, a couple of wards with 10-20 beds, some office buildings and a residence for the doctor. Occasionally there was a simple laboratory capable of basic blood, urine and stool tests. This room would have a few jars of chemicals, some glass slides and a microscope. Sometimes there was an X-ray room used for chest x-rays and looking for fractures, though the machine was frequently out of order. There would usually be a delivery room, very simple but usually the busiest area, and an operating room, but this was often unused. Staff included one doctor, doubling up as public health officer, a couple of Health Assistants (HAs with 3 years training) and Community Medical Assistants (CMAs with 2 years training), plus a few nurses and some cleaners. Sadly, even this skeleton staff could be very inactive, or even absent. There would also be a limited supply of medicines, some out-of-date. The supply from government was small and easily exhausted. This is not meant as criticism, the difficulties were enormous for local staff to overcome and Nepal had severe resource constraints. Over the years there was obvious development, district hospital buildings improved and staffing levels increased. But even 2 or 3 doctors with a team of paramedicals struggle to deal with the health needs of a population numbering hundreds of thousands. They have to deal with an impoverished people prone to natural disasters and diseases. The supply chain and infrastructure will take time to improve.

The camp teams tried to work closely with local health services, communicating with the regional director of health and the district health officers, most of whom were very welcoming. Where possible, they worked alongside local staff and provided maintenance for equipment. Sometimes they had opportunities to teach and train local staff and discussed with staff and patients what to do if any complications arose, and how to communicate with the team. If patients developed problems after the team had left, and needed referral to another centre, the camps would fund that transfer and care. This was very uncommon. Most queries were easily dealt with in discussion with the local medics.

Debra Graumann, an audiologist attending the next ear camp at the district hospital in the hills at Sandhikharka, recollected: "My day started at 7.15 this morning when our hotel owner's son pushed open the bedroom door, announced that he had brought our tea and turned the light on! Now, after 14 hours of almost uninterrupted hearing tests, I'm trying to clear up my room for the next day's work, but patients keep coming, hoping to be seen. The surgeons finished operating shortly after midnight and we headed back to our hotels. There was just a grass mat and a very thin lumpy cotton mattress on my bed. Having sneezed a while at the dust, I finally fell asleep; I was so tired, I slept like a log. My hotel had a shower, a cold tap at shoulder height. I had come with a bagful of hearing aids and the surgeons also gave me more NHS cast-offs. Hearing tests were difficult because of the noise from the crowds in outpatients. I grappled with my few words of Nepali, and when I opened the door for the next patient, half a dozen pushed in and I then pushed them back out. They don't seem to mind! After six days, I became exhausted and asked the driver to take me back to the hotel for a rest and to wash some clothes. I struggled on, to complete my work. When packing up my stuff, I got an electric shock from my tympanometer (a machine for testing middle ear function). The last day we finished early, at

8pm, so that we could all go and have a meal of rice and curry, so nice after chapatis on the run all week. It has been good. I would like to come again. But just now, I want to sleep and eat!"

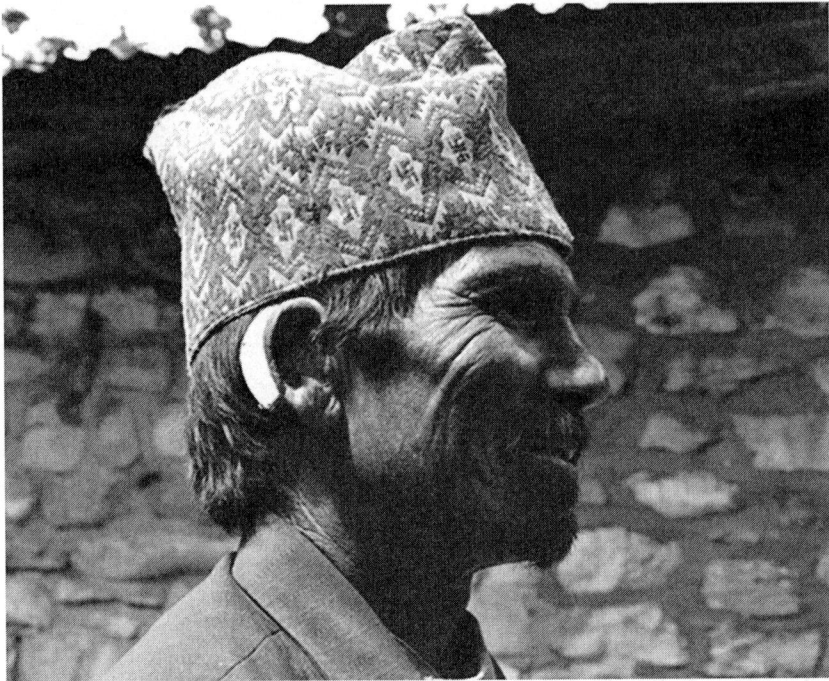

*A village man fitted with a powerful hearing aid for the first time in his life.*

Two weeks after this busy ear camp, many of the same team were off again along the East-West highway, then turning north to Dang Ghorahi, this time with gynaecologists from UK and Australia. The camp followed the well-tested system in the district hospital. INF was well-known in this area, where they had a Public Health team. On one of the evenings at 8 pm, the female patients had begun to line up for the next morning's clinic, to make sure they would get a ticket to be seen. The Maoists arrived, warning the patients that there would be trouble and to take shelter.

At 9 pm, one of the post-op patients collapsed, following a vaginal hysterectomy, and had to be taken back to theatre. She was in a bad way. The battle began to save Suntali. Her blood count was very low; the anaesthetist, when intubating her, said he had never seen a trachea so white. There was no facility for blood transfusion nor for cross-matching blood samples. Radical thinking was necessary if this precious woman was to be saved. On opening the abdomen, much blood was found. With a 50ml syringe, they started sucking the blood out of the abdomen, putting it straight back into the patient's vein via an IV fluid bottle. This was possible as the blood had ceased to clot normally. They continued salvaging the blood whilst finding and tying off the slipped ligature [thread used to tie off a blood vessel]. Her clotting factors had ceased functioning. She was at death's door. A catheter was in place, and her urine was full of blood. It was decided (the nearest hospital being four hours away) to give this bloody urine to her in her IV as every red cell was vital. [I had never heard of this before—Ed]. They needed fresh blood. Ellen and Peter Bisset, an INF member who was stranded in Ghorahi, knew their blood group was O+ve, as did two of the visiting doctors. It was hoped the patient was not Rhesus negative, a 20% risk. The risk of doing nothing was inevitable death. However, there were no facilities for taking blood off into a bag nor the necessary drug (heparin) to stop it clotting. But they had a good supply of syringes.

Ellen was sitting on a box and 20ml syringefuls of blood—the biggest syringe they now had—were taken from her and put straight into the patient. This was repeated time and again. The two doctors gave their blood, and then it was Peter Bisset's turn. Dragged from his bed at 4 am, he also gave blood. Altogether four people gave a total of 1,500mls. Then thankfully, with all these fresh clotting factors in the new blood, her blood began to clot. There was no bad reaction to the blood or the urine. As the blood clotted, there were tears all round.

"I don't believe it. It is not possible. She should be dead," said the anaesthetist, voicing the sentiment of everyone.

Drama enough, but it wasn't finished yet. Ellen, like the others, had worked 20 hours nonstop. She returned exhausted to her hotel, put in her Boots earplugs and crashed out, hearing nothing. The anaesthetist, Joe, and nurse, David Cope, stayed with the patient. Then the shooting began. Bombs exploded. Joe and David hid as best they could until it had finished.

The next thing Ellen heard was a knock on the door. "Oh no," she thought, "the patient has died." Not so. In fact she did well. However, overnight, the Maoists had attacked the army and the police posts in the town. Many were killed. The injured were brought to the hospital where the team was told to keep away, whilst the Nepali doctor did his best. Helicopters took the seriously injured to the Military Hospital in Kathmandu. Ellen and Paul, the other anaesthetist, had heard nothing! Once again, the Maoists had left the medical team and its vehicles unharmed.

Meanwhile, the women who had been waiting to be seen, and the post-op patients, were unfazed by the dramatic events. They pressed the team back to work, tired and shocked as they were. Ellen gave the team the chance to return home, but they chose to stay. The camp carried on until it reached the planned endpoint. 820 ladies were seen and 83 operations performed.

After finishing camp, Ellen spoke to Suntali, "Do you realise you nearly died?" "Yes, I arrived at gates and saw beautiful trees and flowers, but then I heard my children calling for me, so I came back."

There was such a need amongst women with gynaecological problems in Ghorahi that the team returned in April 2002. Suntali returned, very well. How grateful the team was. On the day before they left to travel to Ghorahi, Ellen heard rumours of another fire fight in nearby Dang, where 90 young men had been slaughtered during an attack by the Maoists on the army post. It was thought most of the dead were Maoists. Ellen had wondered about whether to travel but felt it right to continue to Ghorahi, trying to normalise events, and the women came. Rumour had it that there would be another strike lasting several days, so Ellen cut short the camp in order to get the doctors to Kathmandu for their international flights and to send the Nepali team home safely.

There had been a return visit to the ex-Kamaiyas in the Terai in February 2002. Generally, the people looked better than the year before. More houses had been built, and small-scale vegetable crops had been planted. Getting there was potentially hazardous. Halfway, in a remote area with no houses, they had a puncture and were told there was a strike called by the Maoists. Ellen was faced with a difficult decision, as these were dangerous days. The Army offered to go with them, but Ellen thought that was asking for trouble. They went on their own, sailing easily along as there was no other traffic, and arrived with no problem. Other places had not been so lucky. A bus and two lorries had been caught and were burned, as was a bus carrying passengers, all of whom escaped. Fear grew.

During the camp, an army helicopter circled overhead. "I was anxious. The thought of them shooting up the people waiting for treatment was too much for me. In the end, I went out hoping they would see my white skin, red hair and shortish skirt. It worked! They went away."

Ellen tells the story of a 40-year-old woman, blind because of vitamin A deficiency and her boy with a prolapsed iris, preventing him from shutting his eye. "We paid for mother and son to go to the eye hospital." A child of 10 was literally dumped at Ellen's feet. "He can't walk. We have to carry him." In fact, he had one good leg and two good arms and was bright. Ellen showed them how to make crutches from bamboo. He returned in an hour walking with these crutches, beaming all over his face. They were given money to go and buy some proper crutches. They went home with hope. "Who would have thought we would have seen him walking?" said the neighbours.

"When we arrived home, I began to reflect on the wisdom of what we were doing. Was it right to put the lives of others in danger? The Maoists have always looked on us favourably, so we must trust that they continue to do that." Ellen so often found encouragement in her Bible reading, in this case reading from Isaiah "…you will not leave in haste…you will go out in joy." "The battle is not yours but God's."

This was to be another busy year for camps. Despite Ellen's misgivings about the Maoists, having seen the great needs of the neglected hill people, the team pressed on. Next was Baitadi, in the far west, bordering India. The journey took two and a half days in Land Rovers. Wikipedia stated that the district population in Baitadi was 250,000, with 70% living between 3,500 and 9,800 ft, remote and poverty-stricken. I searched for information about communications, and all that was written was about mobile phones, Facebook, etc. No mention of roads or flights! At that time the newly introduced mobile phone network did not extend to rural Nepal, but the team did begin to carry an expensive satellite phone in case of trouble.

One totally unexpected situation arose. A woman arrived in labour with twins, one already stillborn. The local doctor was about to attempt a Caesarian section with little equipment. The team had an anaesthetist and suction, plus dressings. The second twin was also delivered dead, but the woman survived. Ellen had looked on in horror at the beginning, but in the end, the woman said, "If you hadn't been here, I would have died." Following this, the Nepali doctor sought some training in order to cope on his own another time.

Mike and ENT colleagues came from UK to this location. For those for whom it was the first time, it was a great experience and an unforgettable adventure. 'Back-to-back' camps had started. The Nepal-based team would stay for a few weeks. Then visiting teams, typically gynaecology, general surgery, followed by an ear and maybe dental team, would run successive camps. This reduced costs and travel but was very tiring for those away from their homes for weeks on end.

Sarah Caukwell, a British gynaecologist, who later became a consultant in

Plymouth, UK, went on her first camp to Tamghas in Gulmi District. Arriving in Kathmandu, she, with the other doctors, had to register with the Nepal Medical Council "in a shed, with three Nepali professors recounting their training days in UK. They said that this process was required as Indians with no qualifications are setting up as doctors in Nepal." Their journey from Pokhara took four hours on metalled roads and six in four-wheel drive Land Rovers on rough roads "through, round and up mountains, with staggering views as we got higher. Finally, we arrived in Tamghas, a one-street or dirt track town. A policeman had been killed and everyone was appalled." She recalled her first impressions: "Tamghas was pretty gross—one littered dirt track with hovel houses, and open sewers running down the street. Our hotel was revolting; there is no other word for it. We had no water, electricity that lasted a few minutes and then spluttered out for the rest of the day. There was nowhere to sit except broken chairs. The menu had one dish: daal bhat. I managed to live on omelettes and Coca-Cola."

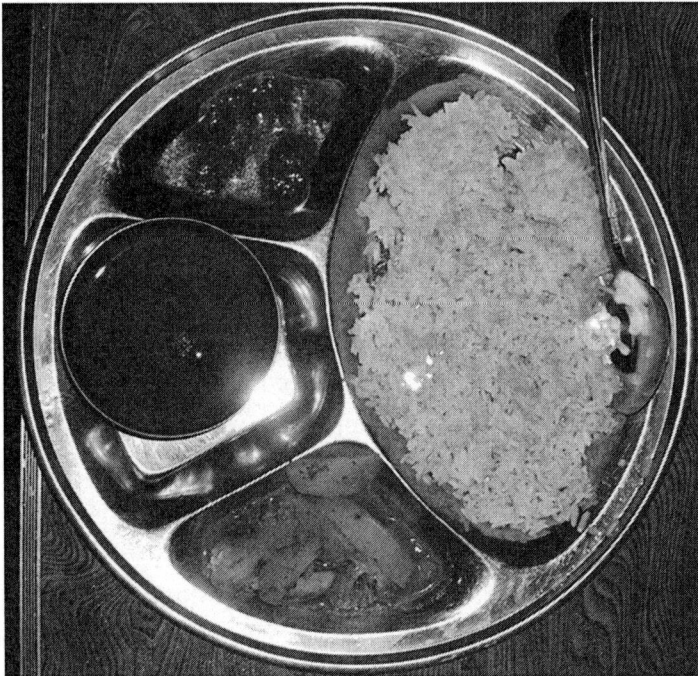

*Standard issue of daal bhat at camp: rice, watery black lentils, vegetable curry and chutney.*

This is a fair expression of the culture shock experienced by many on their first trip to remote parts. Those who live there barely notice these things unless some additional problem or shortage happens! Sarah had some lovely, perceptive insights:

"Ellen, our boss, is a 61-year-old Glaswegian, utterly hysterical, who has been in Nepal for 30 years, spoke Nepali like a native, and took no nonsense from the patients or from us! She is a nurse by training but really manages to be everywhere all the time. She is a truly wonderful person whom we all adore."

She comments on Regina, her Nepali scrub nurse. "She was the most calming scrub nurse I have ever worked with. She would pass me a rusty clamp or a massive needle impossible to use in a vaginal hysterectomy and say, "Sorry, doctor," and I'd just laugh. We loved working with each other, and I would always 'bag' her to assist me if possible.

"At 7:30 am, we would gather for a few songs and a thought for the day and prayers which, surprisingly, I really liked. Then we walked up a hill to the hospital, which we took over and rearranged. We had two simple operating tables (brought by the team), and we sat side by side when operating—a novel experience—and used head torches to see. When we arrived, we saw a queue of women right round the building one and a half times, waiting for us. They had queued all night, and some had walked for days, all dressed in their bright saris. Ellen went along the massive queue, and any lady with her legs spread apart was brought to the front of the queue (we quickly realised that these were the women with massive prolapses), enabling us to start operating on them as soon as possible. Their case notes and their arms were stamped with the same number, so we could follow them through, and they were given a day to come for their operation.

"By the end, I had done more vaginal hysterectomies in a week than I had done in a year at home. I had never operated on such huge and ulcerated prolapses. The greatest problem was keeping the patients warm. We gave each one a blanket and a woolly hat (mostly knitted by volunteers in Wales). Operations were done under spinal anaesthetic, and each was given 1.5 litres of IV fluid. Then post-op, it was up to their relatives to feed them. Ward rounds felt like being in the Crimean War, falling over patients and relatives scattered across the cold floor. I couldn't tell the difference between my patients, but Ellen knew each and every one. Apart from one lady with retention of urine, there were no complications among the 97 we operated on. Four went home with catheters, hopefully for the local healthcare people to remove. Remarkable!"

# Chapter 9

## Transport in Nepal

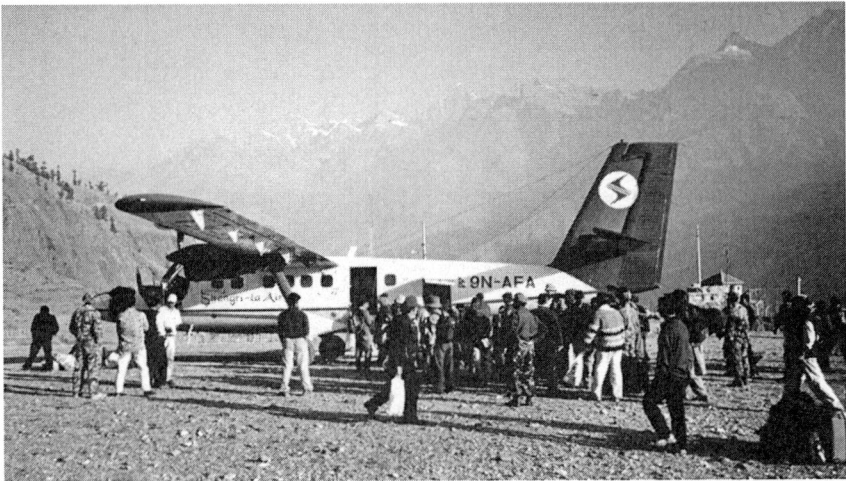

*Team and equipment fly up to Dolpa.*

One of the key elements in the camps in different parts of the western half of Nepal has been the difficulty of getting there and back. Nepal has eight of the ten highest mountains in the world (with 14 peaks higher than 26,250ft). The first range of hills rises suddenly and steeply up to 5,000 ft. Going further north, there are three more high ranges of hills and valleys. Kathmandu at 4,500 ft is in the largest valley, surrounded by 10,000-ft hills. Pokhara is the other major valley, at 3,000 ft. There are high Himalayas, permanently snow-capped, 10 miles from the north end of Pokhara, where the Shining Hospital was built. The Fishtail mountain, 23,000 ft, shaped like a massive Matterhorn, dominates the horizon and is surrounded on three sides by the much higher Annapurnas. At this point in Nepal, the Himalayas come south of the China/Tibet border, and there is a 10-mile strip of high desert land, Mustang, a politically sensitive Tibetan cultural area, north of the mountains.

In Europe, we know how hard it is to cross the Alps. There is hardly a road winding up and over the mountains, which are only half the height of the

Himalayas. It has taken all the ingenuity and engineering knowhow of the Swiss to get through the Alps, and that has been done by building long tunnels.

Europe had enormous communication problems, solved by great engineering. Nepal has not been so fortunate. Whilst it avoided the negative impacts of colonialism, the ruling powers kept the country tight shut to outside influences and opportunities for education and development. There is just one railway in Nepal, across the Terai, crossing the border with India and penetrating 20 miles into Nepal. Whilst Britain was overcoming some of the communication problems in the mountains in northern India, Nepal did not have the means to follow suit. The British built the astonishing 50-mile long narrow-gauge line from Siliguri in the plains up over a 9,000 ft summit, dropping down to Darjeeling and the tea plantations. To the west of Nepal, a railway line was built up to Shimla, India's summer capital in the time of the British Raj, a retreat for the colonial administrators in the Himalayan foothills during the hot season. The politicians of Nepal didn't want any part of colonialism, and development suffered as a result. However, today, China is trying to build a railway line from Lhasa, in Tibet, to the edge of the Kathmandu valley and is heavily involved in attempts to improve the economy, infrastructure and other areas of development in Nepal. A railway line from India into Kathmandu is also being discussed.

Until the 1970s, roads barely existed and, outside a basic system in the Kathmandu valley, there was only one road connection with India, a tortuous, vulnerable road, built in the 1950s. Pokhara had its first connection to the south in 1972 and, a little later, a 130-mile Chinese-built road to Kathmandu. The 500-mile East-West Highway in the Terai was finished around 1980. It was part of a planned but never completed road across Asia to Singapore. These roads were vital for those with access to them. For the rest, it was walking. Gradually, more roads have been built, often starting as dry weather roads with unmetalled surfaces. The torrential monsoon rain has continually washed away bridges and caused landslides on these precariously cut roads on steep hillsides. Bus travel became a vital link as more roads were built, but bus disasters, going over the side and plunging into the rivers below, remain a regular occurrence. These narrow mountain roads are also used by the heavily overloaded Tata lorries, which bring produce from India to the interior, raising living standards. In recent years, the network of unmetalled and metalled roads has developed rapidly, enabling tractors and buses to carry people and goods to almost every district and even to many villages. These roads are fragile and require frequent repair and many can only be used in the dry season. They have led to rapid changes in building techniques (more cement and less local materials) and availability of goods and travel for work and healthcare, if it can be afforded. But in this incredibly steep terrain, people still rely on walking to reach their homes and schools.

Air travel in Nepal is nothing short of amazing. Following the opening of the country in 1951, ex-World War 2 pilots brought their DC3s and ran services to a few grass airstrips. At Pokhara, the tough old DC3s landed on the grass strip, bringing the Nissen huts from Calcutta for the building of the Shining Hospital. Into the 1980s, when a plane left Kathmandu and again as it approached Pokhara, a horn would sound, and people would rush to clear the cows and buffaloes off the strip. People in Green Pastures planning to fly out would wait for those signals and then walk the half mile and cross the deep river Seti gorge and the airstrip to catch the flight. For many years, all internal flights were run by Royal Nepal Airlines, but they eventually became insolvent and a plethora of new airlines sprang up based in Kathmandu. Many of the 75 districts of Nepal gradually built basic airfields. Some are very exciting to arrive at, sometimes with aircraft wreckage at the edges, steep mountains all around and rocky cliffs dropping away at the end of the runway.

The planes used to reach Pokhara were commonly 20-seaters, the Canadian-built Twin Otter being a big favourite, well-tested in the wilds of Canada. In latter days, Dornier, Beechcraft and other 20-seaters or bigger have come in and an international airport is under construction.

Flying in such mountainous terrain needs courage, both for pilots and passengers. For eight months, the weather is generally good for flying, though in Kathmandu, morning fog often disrupts schedules in winter. The four months of monsoon, and the pre-monsoon storms—very violent—make flying uncertain. In recent years, Kathmandu airport has become so congested that there are plans to create other new international airports around the country. If you Google 'The world's most dangerous airports', you will see Nepal with many entries. It is no place to fly in cloud. However, air travel has transformed life for Nepalis, who get subsidised flights, and for tourists, who pay much more. Years ago, I flew from Pokhara to Baglung. It is a 12–15-hour walk. The Twin Otter flight took eight minutes. There was still an easy four-hour walk from the airstrip to Baglung but how much better than walking the whole way! Mountain weather can quickly change. Sadly, but inevitably, there is at least one fatal air crash each year, a very low number, considering the terrain and the many flights. Today, every district has a flight scheduled most days. Air accidents are so few compared with road deaths from cars, trucks and buses crashing down hillsides. Tragically, there have been several international flights lost in the hills around Kathmandu, twice within two weeks in 1999, in fog and low cloud, and once in 2018—an airport accident.

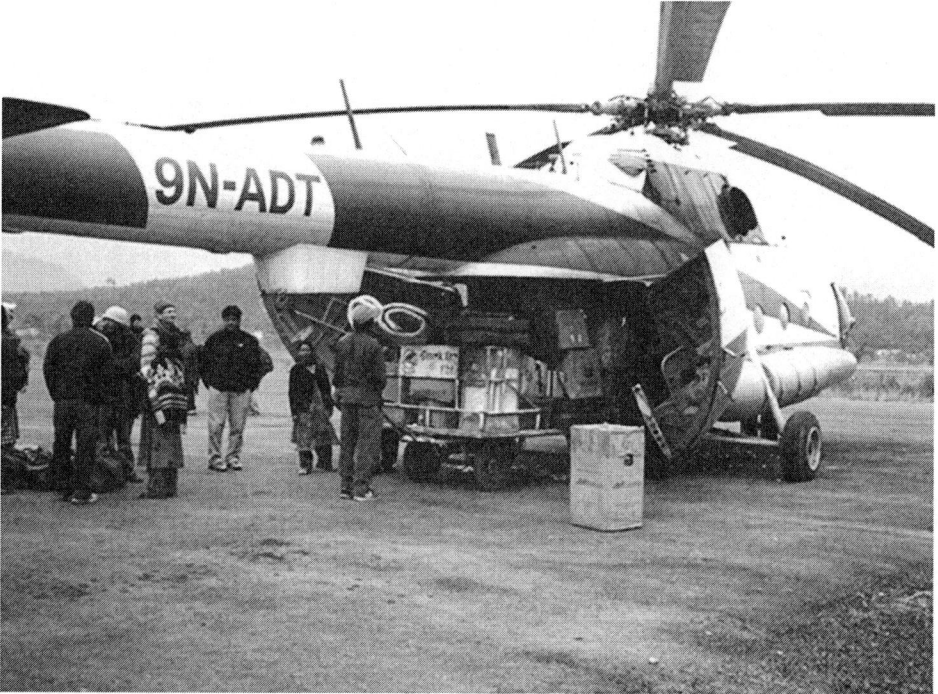

*A heavily laden and elderly helicopter arrives with camp equipment and local supplies.*

Planning for camps always meant working out, not so much where to go—if ease was the criterion, few remote places would ever get any help—but how to get there. To fly from A to B would take an hour, plus walking from the airstrip to the hospital. Taking the Land Rovers—never very comfortable—when Pokhara was the starting point, might involve a two or even three-day drive, with somewhere to stay overnight. That would be OK if there was a fancy Premier Inn or Travelodge. No such luck—very basic 'hotels'. Reasonable for those used to living in Nepal, but all the camps had team members straight from developed countries. Life could be hard for them, even if it was an adventure.

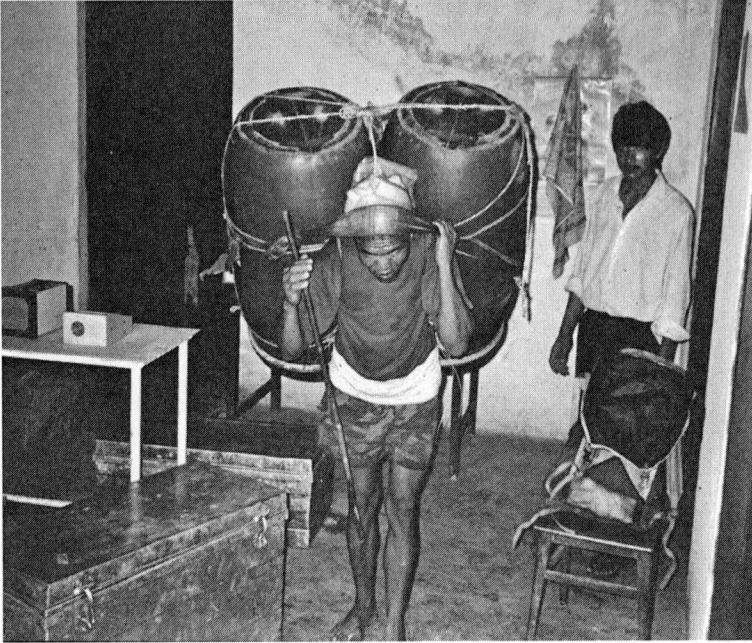

*A porter arrives at a camp in Besisahar before there was a road.*

If, after two long days in a Land Rover, there was then a day's walk, that was hard. Never underestimate walking in the Himalayas. Paths are steep, rough, even dangerous, exhausting in the heat of the day. Don't get ill! There are no toilets. Tummy bugs like amoeba, giardia, bacteria and viruses were common, often from unhygienic food preparation. It is serious stuff. Visiting doctors and other team members fly into Kathmandu. It is easier to fly from Kathmandu to Nepalganj, as few flights go from the camp headquarters in Pokhara unless chartered, which usually costs too much. The roads are extremely tortuous, and many volunteers need to take travel sick pills. Also be ready with pillows for when you fall asleep with head banging against the windows and doorframes as you go over frequent potholes! Road journeys are often interrupted by broken springs, punctures, overheated brakes, and other mechanical issues. Trusting the amazingly resourceful locals is essential. On one journey there was torrential rain and the windscreen wiper motor broke. Mike said, "We tied a long length of string round the wipers then fed it back through the side door on each side and sat and pulled the wipers back and forth for two hours."

# Chapter 10

## The Occasional Camps

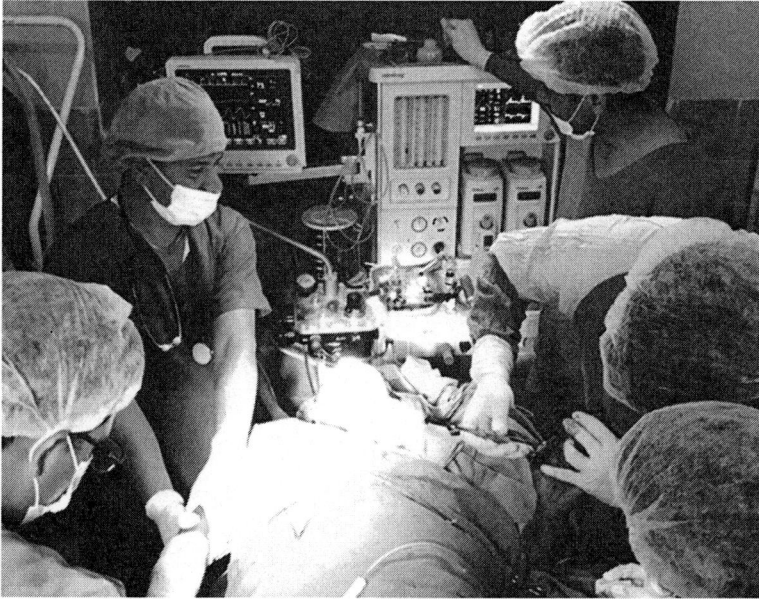

*A surgical team in a peripheral hospital.*

Whilst the great majority of camps were for ear and gynaecology problems and several for surgery and medical treatment, there were a few less common camps. It is absolutely clear that in rural Nepal, there were vast needs, and some patients were so desperate for help that they would walk for days. One man took two aeroplane journeys to find help. The main centres such as Kathmandu, Pokhara, Nepalganj and other cities often had private as well as government hospitals. Pokhara had an Indian medical school, well-equipped and popular, but the villages had nothing. The rural districts might have had hospital buildings, but at this point in its development, the government did not have enough resources to staff and supply them.

Surgery for ears and gynaecology was rarely urgent. Most patients could wait a while and a large, well-equipped team could come with all the gear, and achieve a great deal of work very efficiently in a fairly short time. It was far from perfect, and one hoped that eventually the government system would provide these services. Occasionally, an emergency presented. A moribund boy aged 14 was carried in, pus discharging from his ear. A local doctor told us that his parents had brought him to the hospital earlier and he had stayed several days. It looked certain that he would die, and they had run out of money. "Take him home. An ear doctor is coming soon. If he is still alive, bring him back then", the local doctor told them. After IV antibiotics and resuscitation by the anaesthetists, who worked in an ITU back home, Mike Smith operated, first, on the boy's neck to drain an extensive abscess going down into his chest, then, days later, on his ear, the source of the infection. He had nearly all the possible life-threatening complications of ear disease. In developed countries, this boy would have been in intensive care. When he had recovered enough to stand with help, while dressings were being changed Ellen spoke to him, just as she had to the bleeding gynaecology patient, "Do you realise you nearly died?" "Yes," he replied. "I found myself trying to cross a river, playing beside a big rock. It was lovely. Then I heard my mother crying, so I came back home."

The less common camps were for plastic surgery, dental work and later, specific camps for the gynaecological problem of vesicovaginal fistula. This was socially very debilitating. Obstructed labour could cause a hole to develop between the bladder and the vagina, resulting in continuous incontinence, a rare problem in affluent countries. This could be repaired by specialised surgery, with massive benefit to the woman. Dr Shirley Heywood, a gynaecologist who had previously worked in Papua New Guinea, joined INF and became a member of the camps team. She would later specialise in fistula repair and organise the designated fistula camps. Only 11 patients had operations at the first camp. A year later, 58 operations were performed.

Undoubtedly, general gynaecology camps might try to deal with the problem, but this new super specialisation required specifically trained and experienced clinicians and was very time-consuming. This led Shirley, eventually, to the setting up of a dedicated fistula hospital in Surkhet. In the Shining Hospital, over a period of 25 years, many fistula cases had been operated on by one brilliant general surgeon, Ruth Watson, treating all who came from a wide area. Yet, during these brief visits to village areas in the hills for camps, it seemed as if they could only scratch the surface of need.

Other conditions seen in Nepal included cleft palate and hare lip, which require delicate surgery, often in stages. In developed countries these operations would begin in infancy but in Nepal there were older children and even adults with these distressing and disabling deformities. Burn contractures, resulting from village children rolling into the fire in the centre of their houses, caused permanently bent legs, arms and hands, due to the contraction of scars. It required very precise surgery to protect nerves and blood vessels as the contracture was gradually freed. In this situation and also for acutely burnt children, skin grafting was usually required—quite a dramatic, painful procedure—where, with a special knife, partial thickness skin was taken from an undamaged area and transferred to the area where it was needed. Often the child did not have enough good skin, and a graft would be taken from the mother. This required expertise and there is a risk of the child getting cold whilst exposed and going into shock due to fluid and blood loss. Plastic surgery camps were held in WRH in Pokhara on four occasions, in Nepalganj, twice in Beni and, with quite the biggest attendance, in Rukum. There seemed scope for far more. Ellen recalls one particular patient. "Khim fell off the cliff while cutting fodder for the animals. He fractured his femur and stayed at home till the fracture healed. When he heard we were in the remote area of Musikot, he hobbled for ten hours to get to the camp. Normally, it would take a man three hours to make the journey. We took Khim to Pokhara and paid for his accommodation in the local tea shop until Dr Barat operated to straighten his leg. Khim continued working in the teashop and what money he made, Eka Dev and the shop owner banked for him. When Khim had enough money, he had driving lessons. Then he went to the middle east to make money, came home, and a marriage was arranged. He now has a lovely wife and son and owns a shop. Attending that camp changed Khim's life!!"

One can easily imagine the state of people's teeth in Nepal, without access to dental care and with low levels of fluoride in the water. In some areas, sugarcane is chewed, though few sweets and sugary drinks were available to the poor. However Nepali tea (chiya) is taken very sweet and spicy and often sucked through the front teeth. Dentistry was a Cinderella specialty—in the early days, one of INF's doctors had to go to Lucknow in India for his own treatment. The only treatment in the Shining Hospital years was a shot of local anaesthetic and pulling out the offending tooth—pretty primitive.

Though a full range of treatment was not possible on camps, many teeth were extracted, painlessly filled or cleaned. It was the chance too, for some teaching on dental hygiene.

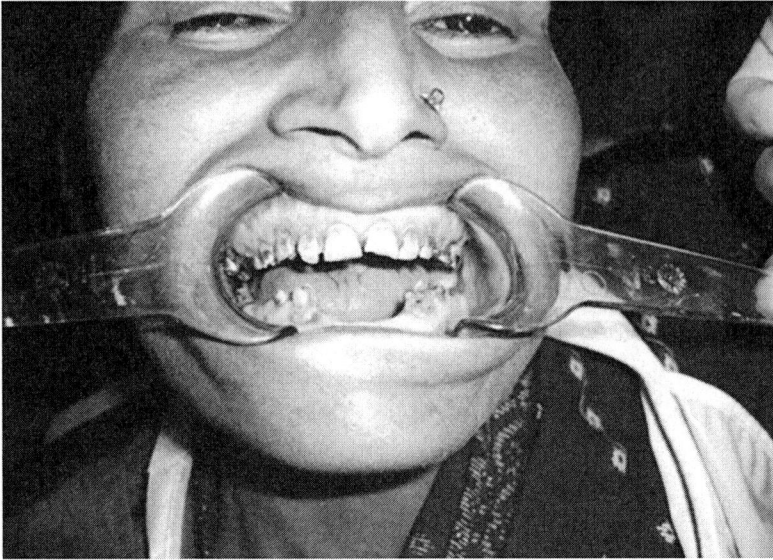

*Tooth decay is common.*

It was also common practice to chew 'pan', a mixture containing tobacco, betel nut and lime, which predisposes to oral cancers. At that time smoking was also widely advertised, though that has now been banned. There were seven dental camps scattered over the 23 years, mostly combined with an ear camp, which worked well.

One was in the village of Tribeni. The team had been invited by local village leaders but they had not realised the logistics. The camp was held in a school, and equipment had to be carried in by porters and mules. The dentist pulled out hundreds of teeth. This camp was in the monsoon, so rain affected the work some days. A huge windstorm caught out some team members as they walked back to the road, when they were crossing a long suspension bridge over the river. Life becomes so difficult if you need to travel in the monsoons.

Another such combined ear and dental camp was held in Arughat one May. Only 91 attended for dental care through the very hot week. In a large marquee, rows of children sat biting on rolls of gauze to stop blood oozing after extractions, whilst cuddling knitted teddy bears provided by elderly ladies in England. The two dentists showed pictures and gave talks on dental hygiene. There was constant amazement that there was no pain. One child came out of the treatment room to an anxious, waiting father. The child was smiling, "I didn't feel a thing. I wasn't frightened."

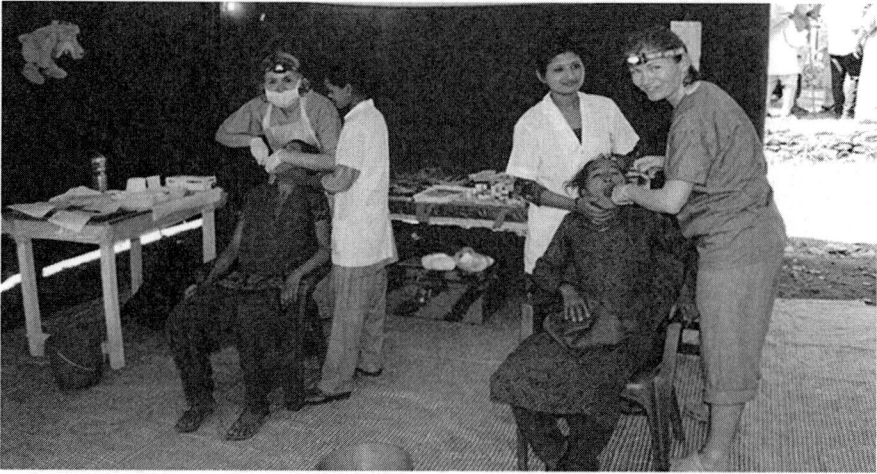

*Dentists Alice and Ros at Arughat camp, doing extractions and fillings and teaching children about dental health.*

Good dentists are invaluable! Most dental camps saw over 300 people waiting for treatment. Alice was Mike Smith's mother's dentist in England. They were chatting about Nepal and Alice's offer to volunteer was quickly accepted! Many volunteers came through similar chance meetings and contacts or recommendations by team members. Mike Smith drew on his large network of ENT contacts.

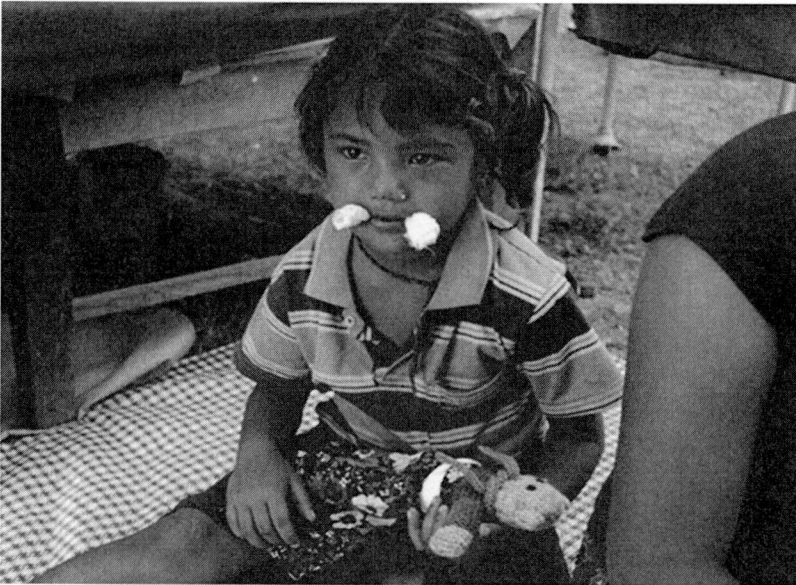

*Child with her teddy bear reward after dental treatment.*

# Chapter 11

## Celebrations

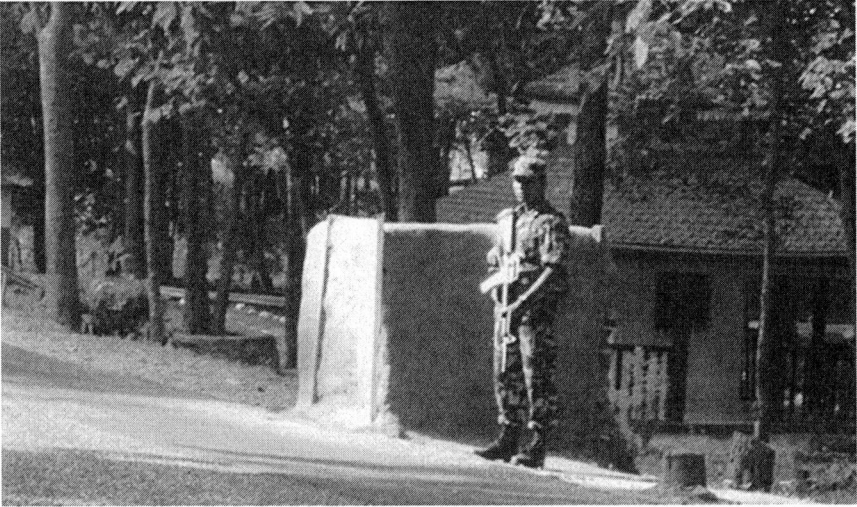

*An Army check-post.*

Following the midsummer monsoon, the busy camps season began again. The first trip was for a five-day medical camp in the heat of the Terai to the ex-Kamaiyas. The hospital in Tikapur was in good order, with caring staff but without a doctor; he had been moved, allegedly for refusing to be involved in corrupt practices. It is hard to be honest in a society where bribery is commonplace. The military were around and Maoist activities never far away. A policeman had been to the camp. He met two people who shook his hand and then shot him dead.

Because of Maoist activity locally, at the last minute Ellen decided to stay at a hotel in the Bardiya National Park. When they arrived, they found a very depressed owner. Because of the political uncertainty, many customers had cancelled their bookings. Very few tourists were visiting Nepal, drastically reducing its major source of income. This poor hotel owner was unable to pay back his loans. The team's arrival was a real blessing to him. At the hotel there were police, drunk in the bar, all carrying guns! Maybe they needed Dutch courage to allow them to cope!

One evening, when the team was returning from working in one of the Tikapur resettlement camps, they passed a checkpoint, usually unmanned. On this occasion, the local Chief of Police stopped them. "Turn everything out," he demanded, "and leave the area." Ellen got out to reason with him—the equipment and drugs had never been subject to a search before. Ellen then discovered that the local 2,000-strong army camp had been bombed the night before. No soldiers had been killed but there was blood on the ground, showing there had been a gunfight with the Maoists. Ellen said she would discuss moving hotel with the team but told him, "We only fear God, not the Maoists or the police." At that point, he gave up, did not search the vehicles and troubled them no more! On the way home, one heavily laden Land Rover broke down. Fortunately, another was available, and it towed the broken vehicle 10 hours back to Pokhara, an exhausting end.

This was followed by a four-day dental camp in the wildlife park, with 223 people treated. A very busy time for the dentists! A month later, a medical camp was held there and in between, a return visit to Baitadi for a gynaecological camp. This got off to a slow start. It seemed that the women were waiting until the team were on site, then, by the end of the second day, they were overrun! It was humbling that some women had travelled for four days to get the help they needed. The woman who had had the Caesarian Section at a previous camp turned up. She was well. Other patients from previous camps also reported good results. Feedback is very encouraging. Baitadi had had a special place in the heart of Dr Pat (Lily) O'Hanlon, founder of the mission. Although it is unlikely that she ever visited before retiring in 1968, she would have been delighted that these camps were held there.

"We weren't often stopped by the police or army, but after an ear camp in the far west, there was a long queue of vehicles, including very fancy vintage Sunbeams, Mercedes open top sports cars, Bentleys, etc. They were on a Himalayan car rally! Our camps co-ordinator Eka Dev Devkota came up to our vehicle. 'We have to wait till the Maoist army officers give their speeches.'" Ellen was not for that!

"I jumped out of the vehicle and went to the man with the microphone in his hand: 'We have just come from an ear camp in Doti and want to get to Nepalganj. We have foreigners who need to catch their flights. Please let us through.'

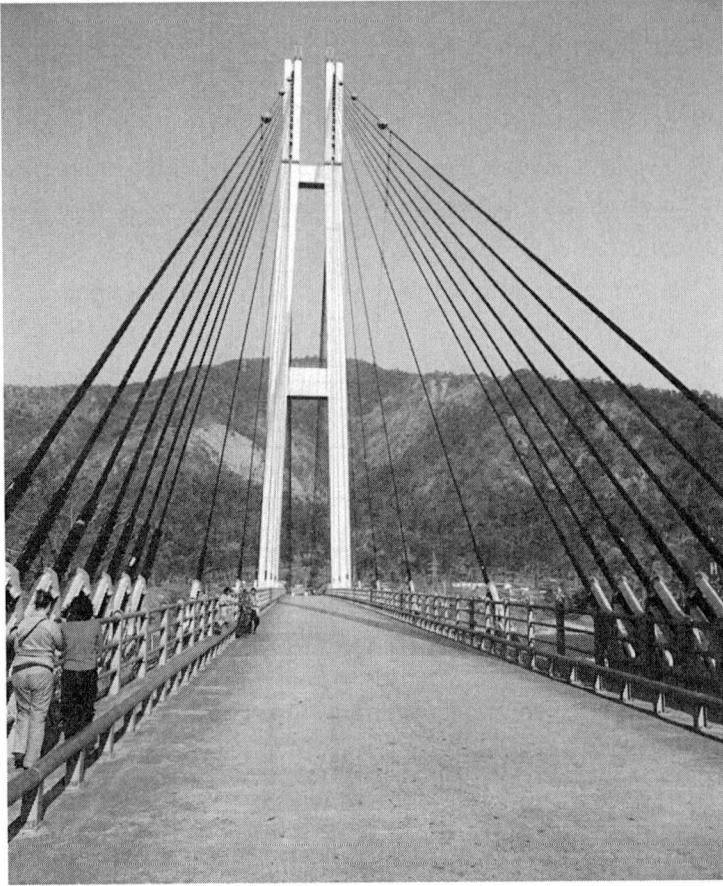

*The bridge over the Karnali river in western Nepal, site of the Maoist army roadblock.*

"They conferred with each other, then waved us through. The poor car rally folk tried to follow us but were not allowed to move." Mike had a different perspective: "I think the Maoist commander was more frightened of Ellen than we were of them." Many of the uniformed Maoist soldiers were very young teenagers.

Then came the first celebration. It was 50 years since the first missionaries had been allowed to enter Nepal. Much had changed. The Shining Hospital had merged into the Western Regional Hospital, and community outreach had brought significant improvement in the villages. TB was being more effectively treated, and leprosy was coming under control through the TB/Leprosy programme. Green Pastures, the original leprosy hospital, continued, but increasingly, it was now used as a rehabilitation centre for many additional types of disability. Soon it would become the centre for treating and rehabilitating those unfortunate people with spinal fractures and injuries (some as a result of the civil war), bringing hope to those paraplegics, who had been the family wage earners, but were now immobile and incontinent, condemned to lie dying slowly of infection and bedsores if they could not find help.

"The Jubilee conference was especially nice for the 1970 group, as most of us managed to attend. How our chins wagged as we went down memory lane. How good to meet up with folk who had walked the same paths over the years." For Ellen, it was a great time spent with the 'class of 1970' with whom she had learned the language and culture and begun work. This time of great encouragement, in the lovely month of November, was followed by two more camps before the Christmas holiday. She had planned another trip to the hills, but elections were due, so it could have been a time of heightened tension. Therefore, they decided to hold the ear camp in the WRH in Pokhara, under Mike Smith's care. They were allowed first use of the brand new operating theatre. For Ellen, it was good to be in her own bed, but her hips and legs suffered from climbing the hospital stairs, until she had to stop. Arthritis was beginning to trouble her.

Christmas Day was spent at one of the Nepali churches. It is always an amazingly well-attended day in this predominantly Hindu country, and 600–700 people attended this service, followed by a 'Love Feast'. During the service, which regularly lasts three hours, a team kills several goats and prepares rice and curry for the meal, eaten sitting cross legged on straw mats laid out in the sun. All are invited to join in, regardless of caste or religion.

On New Year's Eve, Ellen was in the office preparing for the next camps when the telephone rang. "Is that Ellen Findlay?" "Yes. Who wants her?" "This is the British Ambassador in Kathmandu." "Oh yes, and I'm Mickey Mouse. Who is it?" "No, really, I am the Ambassador and I am phoning to tell you that you have been awarded an MBE by the Queen in her Honours List, for outstanding service to Nepal through health and development work!" Ellen was shocked. Very appropriately, her efforts had been noticed. She was 60 and had been working in Nepal for 32 years. The National English medium newspaper, Nepal News, reported the event. She was able to receive her award on a visit to Britain later, from Prince Charles in Buckingham Palace, an honour for the INF team as well as Ellen. The busy year of 2002 finished with celebrations.

# Chapter 12

## Desperate Poverty

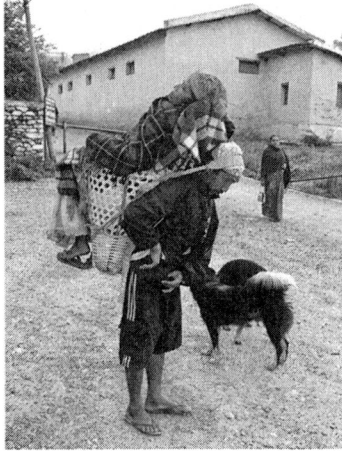

*Patient transport in remote Gulmi.*

Before setting off for the first camp in the New Year, a gynaecology camp, Ellen had been reading the Bible, as was her daily habit. She read, "My eyes are fixed on you, O Sovereign Lord; in you I take refuge—do not give me over to death". This verse was to come to mind more than once, to encourage her during the hazardous days ahead!

Tamghas, in Gulmi District, was up in the hills, a long drive for the medical team, along with the regular Nepalis, led by Eka Dev, who had developed a remarkable and dedicated camps team. These people were all part of Ellen's and Eka Dev's responsibility.

Gulmi District, with a population of 290,000, was renowned for its oranges and coffee, and cobalt could be mined there.

The journey began fairly comfortably on metalled roads, then turning north, they headed into the hills. The road is cut into the hillsides, climbing up, then winding down, uncomfortably narrow, with evidence of landslides, still treacherous, and big drops down to the river below. "It is always good to arrive! The accommodation was atrocious and expensive for Nepal. The rooms were so damp. And it was cold. I didn't have a proper wash throughout my time there." If that was Ellen's experience, it must have been dire for the visitors!

The day before the team's arrival, there had been a battle, just six miles away. The dead from the security forces were being brought into town by helicopter. The next day, a ceasefire was agreed, and the place became less tense. The hospital was in a poor state. "They knew we were coming, but the place was dirty, the staff lethargic and unhelpful. The sinks hadn't been cleaned in years, with red betel juice spit in them. We had to sweep the floors and remove the detritus of a Family Planning clinic that had been held there 10 days previously. Perhaps part of our work was to clean up local hospitals! It is easy for the local staff to get demoralised, but it really comes down to leadership."

Claire Ferrer (nee Stevens), now a GP in Derbyshire, later wrote to Ellen: "We have so many good memories of camps it's difficult to put them all into words. I would like to thank you for inviting Ian and me on these camps, which played a large part in our family lives and the direction our life has taken. They served to keep us humble, aware of the huge need and contrast with our own country and work in General Practice. They enabled us to stay connected with a country still so close to our hearts.

"I remember one of my first camps in Musikot, Khalanga. We flew into this remote village and landed on the field that served as an airstrip. It was the middle of the Maoist uprising and as we landed, with some apprehension, we found the whole plane surrounded by men pointing guns at us! Fortunately, they were the Nepali army troops, there to protect us, but that also made us something of a target for the Maoists. In fact, we were left undisturbed by the Maoists, but one day the camp and village were very quiet and subdued. One of their own young men had been killed and his body was returned for cremation. We watched across the silent village as smoke spiralled up from the funeral pyre.

"It was a good walk up the hill to the hospital. This was a welcome break before sitting in a dark room with newspaper at the window, seeing patients for the rest of the day. Nepalis were very inquisitive and would find any chink to peer through the window at the patient I was consulting, difficult when this involved a gynaecological examination! A thin curtain, sheet or often just a newspaper pinned over the window was important.

"We stayed in a large lodge with more beds than rooms and all the women on camp slept in one room, with just enough space to tuck our luggage under the beds. We had some atypically strange, puzzled, and sometimes quite hostile looks from the villagers, and washing outside at the village tap in the morning made me feel very uncomfortable! The lady of the house ran a tight ship and would wake us all up very early in the morning at about 5 o'clock. Together with the cockerels crowing, she made it impossible to sleep any longer.

"When our hostess decided to come for a hysterectomy at our camp, we sighed with relief; we all had more rest than ever before, and post-op she started to talk about life in her lodge. It was apparently a large brothel, which we had taken over! No wonder we had some strange looks! She talked about how easy it was to spot the women who had earned money in the house, as they would often appear in new saris. I loved the bright, colourful sari fabrics and had just bought one, so I was teased for the rest of the camp! Often the queue for our outpatient clinic was a stunning sight; beautiful women in rich red and gold saris, dressed in their best outfits to see the doctor.

"I had Pratibha Manaen as a translator for that camp, and many times I would find her in tears: 'I never realised people lived like this,' she said. She had lived in Kathmandu all her life and had no idea of life in remote areas. This changed her life and she has written about it since. I had the pleasure and privilege of meeting her many years later in Pokhara. She spoke of her time in camp as very significant in her life. A Nepali gynaecologist came on the camp team this time and looked astonished at our delight at walking up the hill in the morning; 'Do you walk like this in your country?' she asked. She also had lived most of her life in Kathmandu."

Patients poured in for the ear camp in Khalanga, the centre of Rukum. Many were low caste, very poor and in desperate need of medical care. People with lice, worms, and very dirty, with many skin infections, were all treated. Cleaning out ears, they found several with flies in the ear, one with four, which were washed out by syringing. One man, from the Tibetan border, had to be given money for his hotel and air fare, and also a warm sweater. He commented, "You have given so much. What love!" Another man had had ear infections for many years. He wept, "You people are like gods to me. I never thought I would have an operation on my ear." "We knew we were nothing of the sort but had talents and opportunities given us by God and we wanted to use them for good." A well-dressed young man came. He introduced himself by saying, "I am a Maoist. Thank you for caring for my ear. Will you do the same for other Maoists? We know the work you people are doing and you have no need to be frightened of us. We will not harm you." It was so good to be reassured again, because Ellen,

Mike and Eka Dev felt very responsible for the team and the volunteers. Team members sometimes became ill or needed help and support. Eka Dev recalled that Mike was ill one day with a bad migraine and vomiting. Fortunately, the next morning he was fit to do a mastoidectomy as usual.

A father brought his son saying, "My son's tongue doesn't work properly". It was true; the boy was deaf and so spoke poorly. There was nothing wrong with his tongue, the problem really was that he could not hear well enough to imitate speech sounds correctly. He was terrified of having a hearing test, or of anyone going near him. Somebody had brought toys, and Amor was given several small cars to play with. Then he was happy to have a hearing test. He was so different after having a hearing aid fitted. He could hear better for the first time in his life. It would open the door to education in days ahead. Seemingly simple, small and easily fitted, yet actually sophisticated equipment made such a difference. While the surgeons were treating, often curing, persistently running ears, and saving some from brain abscesses, others were syringing ears and fitting hearing aids. Long term maintenance of aids and supply of batteries was an ongoing concern, and time was spent counselling each patient about how this could be achieved. The future of this service was frequently discussed, and this led to several research projects.

On the last morning, while they were changing dressings and giving instructions to the patients, another well-dressed man with a swollen hand was standing around. The team looked at it and cleaned it and treated him with antibiotics. His response? "I'll never forget you for helping me like that. This hospital is rubbish!" It turned out that he was a member of the hospital committee!

It wasn't long before the next camp, in mid-March, was taking shape. Maoist activity had increased along the East-West Highway, with multiple road blocks. It was therefore decided to go to Dolpa by air, though finances were low. There was no scheduled flight from Pokhara, so a 20-seater plane was chartered. The price was $3,000, "More money than we had in the bank." Ten minutes later, the agent phoned back: "You have a lot of people and luggage. You will need two planes, costing $6,000." "I felt sure that it was still right to go". The team were flown in, followed by a three-hour downhill walk with all the equipment to the government hospital.

The area is remote, arid and beautiful, at about 7,000 ft, surrounded by high mountains and near the famous blue Phoksundo lake. The people up there are very poor. Very few vegetables grow on the rocky ground. The cattle have hardly any grass to eat and so give very little milk. Every year, the government of Nepal flies thousands of kilos of rice in to help the people survive the bitter winter.

The camp was being held in the Health Centre, in Dunai, Dolpa district. Once again, the Nepali doctor, Purusotam Raj Sedain, was extremely helpful. For some, accommodation was provided close to the hospital, whilst others had a 20-minute walk to their hotel. Locals helped with translation and organisation. One of the surgeons was Carl from the north of England. When Mike met him at Heathrow airport, knowing what was ahead for them, he was amazed to find him in smart black city shoes, Mackintosh coat and a trilby hat! Carl shared a very basic room with Mike and Charlie Collins. The walls were made of crude planks nailed side by side. Carl would carefully wash and hang out his Y fronts each morning, providing much amusement, which he took well!

This was a seven-day camp. Patients were slow to arrive at first. Probably they wait to see if the team will turn up. They have been let down before, though not by the camps team. Work had to finish by 6.30pm, to beat the curfew. One patient walked for 10 days for his surgery, very hard for us to comprehend. 689 patients were seen and an amazing 325 of them had audiology tests, resulting in 54 hearing aids being fitted. The surgery performed was complex, mainly ear drum and mastoid operations, but two patients had deafness caused by fixation of the stapes in the middle ear, the smallest bone in the human body. Delicate operations (stapedotomy) were performed to remove and replace the tiny bone, restoring their hearing. A few children were fitted with grommets.

Sandra Chinnery, an Austrian nurse and INF member, who joined the camps team many times, described her experience: "It was a real privilege for me to take part in this camp. The team was accommodated in three little hotels. Our 'shower' was a tap beside the footpath into town. Every day we ate our rice in a small, smoky kitchen. Through the smoke it was nearly impossible to see anything, nor to taste much, but it was probably better that way!

"One day we were part of a miracle! The lady who cooked our daily meal had a son. When he was four years old, he had had very severe meningitis, which led to complete hearing loss. The parents had taken him to Kathmandu and Nepalganj to have him examined, but every time they got the same answer: 'Sorry, nothing can be done. Hearing aids will not work, because of his extreme deafness.' Very pessimistically, his mother brought him to our doctors for one last hope. Suddenly, the audiometer showed a trace of hearing in one ear!

Fortuitously, our audiologist, Laura, prior to leaving her office at home, had picked up a high-powered hearing aid from the drawer. This was fitted and Biswas could hear some sound for the first time in 12 years. It made his face shine! We were all very moved."

Laura wrote after the camp: "It was by far the most adventurous and challenging trip that I have ever had the privilege of being involved with. Things are really put in perspective, such as the last time you had a bath, the last time you ate anything other than rice and curried vegetables and the last time you were anywhere with reliable electricity."

Ellen remembered another patient: "A young man had arrived too late for the ear camp in Jumla, three years previously, travelling for days from his home in Surkhet. He heard we were coming to Dolpa, so he took two flights to get to us. He got his surgery. We were amazed that he had enough confidence in us to go to such great lengths to get help."

The three hour walk back up the mountain to the airstrip was steep and hot in the bright sun. Nevertheless, Sandra started off up the slope, despite being heavily pregnant. Ellen, meanwhile, came on a pony, to the team's delight! As Sandra continued to struggle on, finding it hard to catch her breath and tired at the end of camp, someone procured a mule for her too. This was a mixed blessing! She had never ridden a horse before and found it scary, added to which the mule insisted on walking far too close to the edge of the precipice.

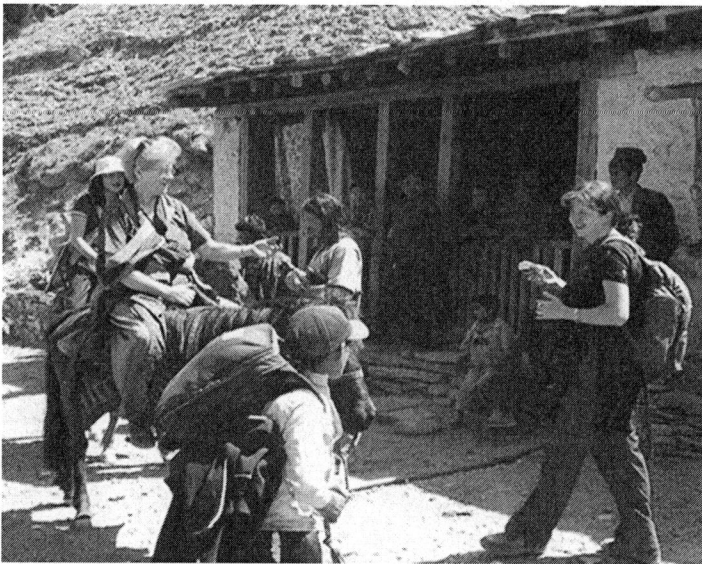

*Ellen riding to Juphal airstrip in Dolpa.*

93

If patients needed further surgery, they were told where and when future camps would be held. Communications were improving. Not only were camps announced on local, and sometimes national radio, even in remote villages, people began to own mobile phones. It became possible for them to phone the central office in Pokhara for information. Pathology reports could be emailed to surgeons in their home countries for decisions to be referred back to Nepal.

Ellen had known that this camp would be very expensive to run, using chartered flights. As she walked along the path with Ann Dingle (an ENT surgeon and one of the most regular camp volunteers), Ann said, "We should send a proposal to the British Medical Association, they have recently advertised a £2,000 grant." Ann made the application and we got the money!! Ellen wrote: "On returning back to my home in Pokhara, once again, a whole host of gifts were awaiting us. Sally and Stafford had a 40th wedding anniversary and asked friends to send money to camps instead of gifts. This made up the shortfall."

Travel in Nepal in May (pre-monsoon time) can be very unpleasant, with uncomfortably hot days, especially at low altitude. Evening is usually better, with a breeze. The camp team was off again, firstly driving to Nepalganj. It was a journey Ellen remembered vividly: "We felt we were travelling in a hot oven, and temperatures reached 43°C. Such was the heat that we each drank four litres of water. From there the plan was to fly the 20 minutes into Rukum airport, but the plane only went on a Wednesday!" They chartered a flight, with the promise that a plane would be available to fly them back out. "The Chaujhari hospital was the busiest hospital we have been in; it was formerly run by the United Mission to Nepal (UMN). There was a very good atmosphere. They told us it would take us 30 minutes flat walking to reach our hotel. Hmm. In fact, we dropped 200 feet and then climbed up 600 ft on a 40-minute walk!" Not ideal in the heat and after a full day's work.

This was Dr Shirley Heywood's first camp. She was still doing her first year of language study and this made for excellent language and culture training. She didn't think much of the hotel, with five to a room. Rumour had it that it was usually another brothel! It had one toilet, and the tap was in the street—not so good for washing. The walk to the hospital involved crossing two small rivers— much better for a wash! Curfew was in place, but the team worked late. Ellen informed the police and asked them not to shoot at the people returning with their headlamps shining.

"A young girl came. She hoped to marry but she had a large fibroid uterus.

She had been to several centres but each one had said 'you need a hysterectomy'. David, one of the Ipswich gynaecologists, thought it might be possible to preserve the girl's uterus. As often happened when there was difficult surgery, the surgeons operated while the rest of us prayed. When I returned to Rukum later, the girl's brother came down to tell me that his sister had married and now had a baby."

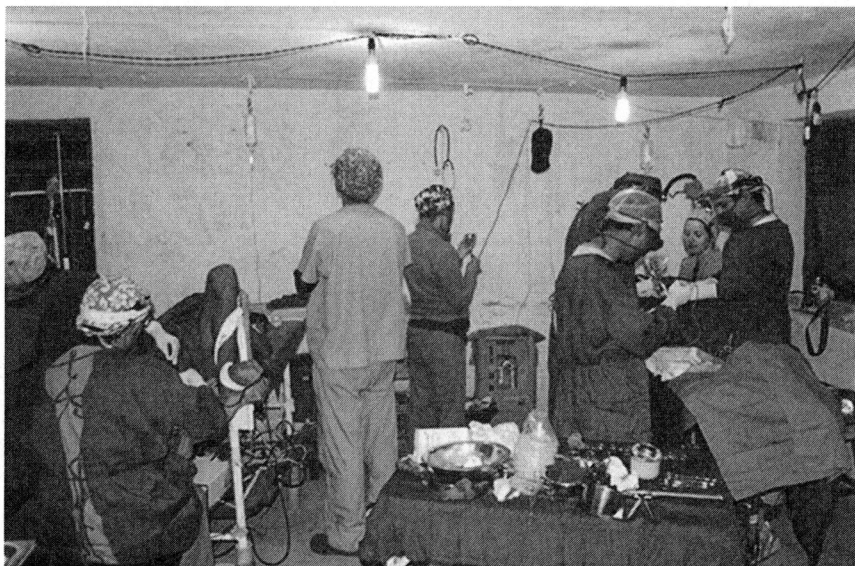

*A surgical camp, operating room.*

Now there were two more camps to prepare, a gynaecology camp in October and an ear camp in November. Both of these were to be in Rukum in the heart of Maoist controlled areas, but with no fighting now. For the ear camp, they managed to rent two very basic houses near the hospital, avoiding the 40-minute walk from the district centre town of Khalanga to the small local hospital, allowing more time with patients, and being nearby in case of any complications at night. There were no beds, bedding or shower. Some of the team slept on mud floors. In the night Maoist troops could be heard marching through the village. There was water. Washing was at the village pump. But at least the toilets were clean, a hole in the ground, a bucket of water, woven bamboo walls, and sacking for doors. They really were camping!

Mike paid a courtesy visit to the Chief District Officer in the village centre. This meant walking along a twisting path between rolls of razor wire, overlooked by sandbagged military emplacements, and soldiers equipped with old rifles. The poor CDO seemed completely isolated in his compound. We were told that the whole district, outside this centre, was controlled by the Maoists. Electricity was a problem initially. Our generator was carried time and again to the camps, with fuel, which allowed the operating microscopes to be used. An elderly lady came with her family, she had a goat bone stuck in her throat. In Nepal meat is usually chopped into pieces with a traditional Nepal knife (Khukri) and stewed. Everything is included and nothing wasted, bone, skin, gristle. She had a large sharp bone lodged in her upper gullet. Mike and Alan Johnson (a surgeon from England) struggled to dislodge it, but eventually Alan succeeded. The bone had been stuck for some days, so she needed a drip and tube feeding while she recovered, sitting cross legged on a mat in the sun each day.

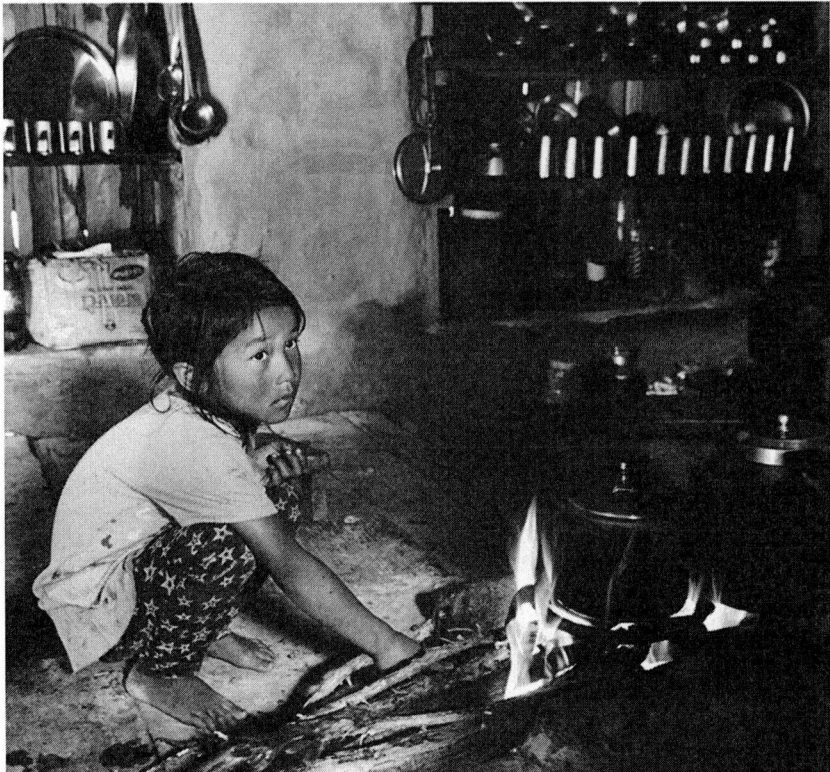

*Young girl cooking over an open fire in Rukum.*
*Photo: Aaditya Chand*

Rukum was—with Dolpa, Doti and Rolpa—the heartland for Maoist recruitment and activity. In later years, after peace was established, a walking trail in this area of lakes and marvellous scenery was called Guerrilla Walk.

Police were everywhere in town, though not in the hospital. Some post-op patients were terrified to be there at night. There were bad stories. One complete village had been driven out, taking nothing with them. Their savings in a local bank were also stolen. One frightened man was with his son. The other half of his family were in his village, but he could not return there. A deaf mute 16-year-old girl came; her mother was begging for the girl to be sterilised. She had had a pregnancy aborted (illegal in Nepal) and was at risk of repeated rape. "The Maoists have stabbed my husband and son to death," her mother said.

Six-year-old Loti was carried in a doko (basket). She was badly burned, and smelly because of infection. Her father couldn't afford to spend money on Loti so we asked him to take her to Pokhara (they came back in the vehicle with us) and he stayed with her for eight weeks. The camps team took responsibility for her, ensuring she had food, clothing, etc. After multiple surgeries, Loti recovered and went home healthy. Many years later she phoned the office to say she had passed her SLC (School Leaving Certificate) exams and was now married.

Inevitably, there was much poverty. A man walked a whole day to sell his potatoes. He heard his wife could have family planning, so rushed home, bringing her back and also another couple. They had £2.00 between them for food. The wives were sterilised and needed a couple of days rest. They then had nothing. Ellen decided to support them from the poor fund. "We gave them a Rs500 note (£5.00). They looked at it, turned it over and over. 'Do you know what that is?' Eka Dev asked them. They had never seen one before, so we swapped it for smaller denomination notes, to their delight."

200,000 people live scattered through this district, almost all in the steep hills and valleys high on the slopes of Mt. Dhaulagiri. Survival is a struggle, even without a civil war. The local people were delighted that two months running, camps had come to Rukum. The hospital Medical Superintendent was rarely there; he was either on courses or holiday or seeking a post in Kathmandu! The owner of a local teashop said to Ellen, "The people in Kathmandu do not know that Rukum exists. They have forgotten all about us." On the whole, Nepalis are frightened to come to Rukum and who could blame them? Yet the INF medical team frequently went there and brought relief to some and hope to many more. These were desperate days in Nepal.

The promised two planes to fly the team out were commandeered by the military and, though some caught a flight, Eka Dev and others had to walk. The

97

baggage, requiring five porters, was carried for 10 hours in the heat to the road head.

Five days after finishing the ear camp, Ellen left her home in Pokhara to return back to her flat in Scotland, waiting for the next phase of life to be revealed.

# Chapter 13

## A Surgical Patchwork

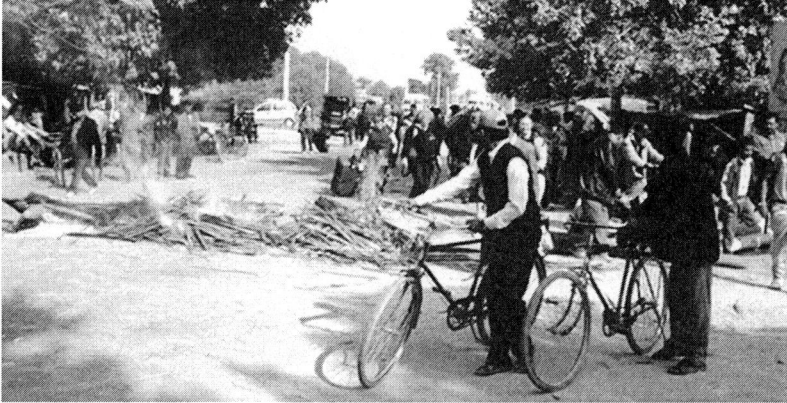

*Crossing a roadblock near Nepalganj in the Terai.*

Although, for the most part, Ellen Findlay seemed to sail through these many camps in truly remote locations with few complaints, she is only human! Being in Nepal for 30 years had enabled her to experience the extremes of climate, the problems of transport and Nepali customs and cultures. There were times when they threatened to overwhelm her: dirty hotels, smelly toilets (if present!), careless rural hospital staff, filthy hospitals. The long journeys took their toll. As she got older, Ellen's hip joints frequently caused pain, especially when walking for hours on rough, steep and dangerous paths. Her stamina was enormous. Her sense of purpose—to help the poor and forgotten people of rural Nepal—drove her on. She loved these people, and they loved her.

We get a glimpse of the inner strains and resources in a letter home in 2003:

"Do you ever have a week you would like to re-live and hope it was better than before? I've just had one of those weeks. Though our last gynae camp was busy and positive, some news was not positive. That put me in the depths of despair for a couple of days. I almost bought a one-way ticket out of Nepal, deciding I would never return. As usual, the Lord and friends got me over the bad patch.

"Then a few of us went down with sore throats and aches and pains. I got over that, and then a bug hit. Then when my house water supply dried up, despair hit again. I visited a cancer patient, and she said she would get a tank of water for me. That lifted my spirits again."

Her mood was not improved when the team returned from Pyuthan in the hills on the great festival day of Holi. Why did they do that? Red dye is liberally thrown everywhere and anywhere. "Sometimes fun, but often threatening, with drunkenness and highway robbery! Before letting the vehicles pass, they demanded anything from Rs1 to $100. I felt I couldn't face another journey on the road again. The next camp was to be in Dolpa. The thought of 12 hours in the vehicles, then a one-hour flight, followed by a three-hour walk to the ear camp was too much." The Maoists were escalating their attacks and disruptions as they sought radical change.

"There are roadblocks everywhere. The main towns have a police and army presence, but in between, the Maoists rule. For us to attempt the 12-hour journey to Nepalganj, we would have to pass through four districts. The risks to life and limb are too great. Vehicles are being torched, tourist vehicles burnt. On a previous occasion, we hadn't wanted to disappoint the people in Dolpa and had chartered a plane. This time, we decided to go somewhere cheaper. We later heard that the government was running a camp in Dolpa at just that time, so we could not have worked there anyway."

The visa situation in Nepal was bringing change. All expatriates who had been in Nepal on work visas for ten years or more would not get their visas renewed. This would affect many of the NGOs (non-governmental organisations) who had worked for many years helping build up the country. These were the people with the best contacts, most experience and best language skills. It was hard to comprehend this government policy. Projects created many local skilled jobs. This, of course, affected Ellen. Most of her team, outside the volunteers, were employed by the charitable organisation and were Nepali, well-led by Eka Dev. Even before this change, Ellen had been wondering about leaving Nepal, and on her previous return from the UK, had not brought as many supplies as usual—clothes and dried food were a normal accompaniment to supplement the goods in the shops, especially when visiting the villages and rural areas.

Her preparedness made clearing up her affairs more leisurely than for most. A big concern was for the welfare of her house girl, Anju, who had worked for her for 14 years and would be unlikely to find a similar job. Six other mission staff were also forced to leave.

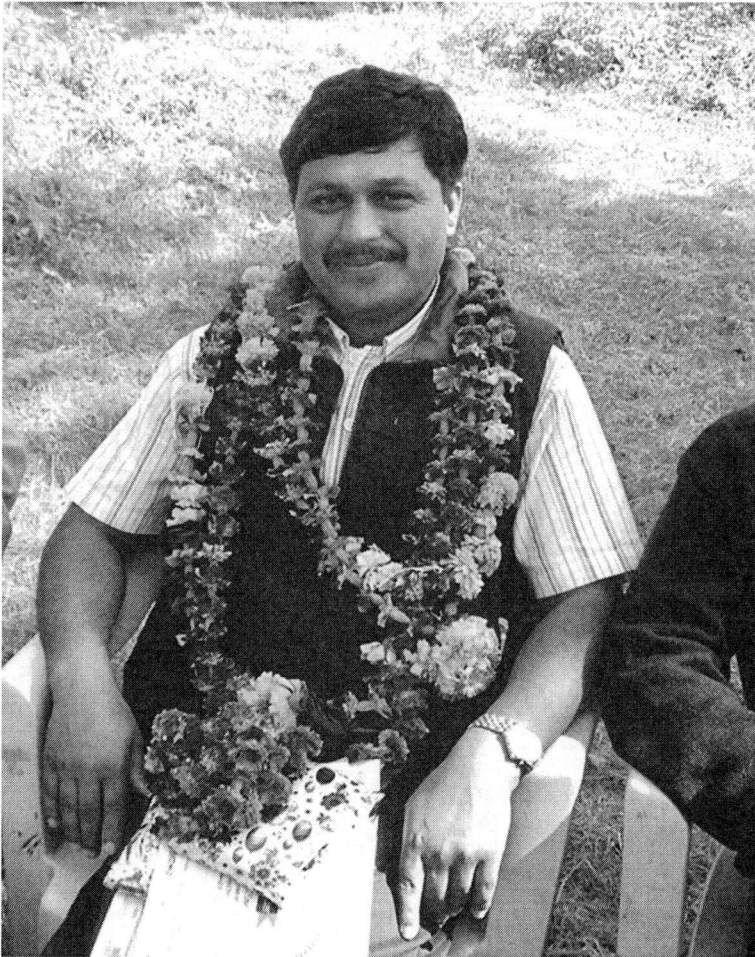

*Eka Dev Devkota, invaluable camps co-ordinator.*

Fortunately, INF had run a small pension fund for the workers, so Anju would get some money. Out went the books and clothes; accounts at home and in the office were made ready. The Nepali camps staff were upset, having worked so long under Ellen's leadership. Communication and fundraising could be difficult. Most difficult of all was leaving her old dog, Rags.

All these visas ended that year on December 5th. "Though I'm not so young, I'm too active to retire." People had offered to petition the government, even the King. Ellen felt that it was the time to leave but wanted to continue to come back on tourist visas, which allow a maximum of five months each calendar year in Nepal.

What was the purpose in refusing to renew the visas of long-serving workers? It didn't prevent them returning, to continue their work on tourist visas, but they were restricted to five months per year. It was a major disruption for families with children at school, requiring big decisions. For people committed to long-term work, building something significant for the Nepali community, returning home and finding other work produced a crisis. On the positive side, it resulted in Nepalis already working in projects taking over from their expatriate bosses in part or whole, a move necessary for the building of a strong, independent Nepal. A decade later, Nepal took the next step, requiring all projects to be Nepali led, with only expatriates with Masters degrees or equivalent given work visas. INF already had this process in place.

For camps, this meant that workers such as Eka Dev now had greater responsibility in management. For Ellen, in practice little changed, he was already running things efficiently.

"This semi-retirement mode I am now in could spoil me for life. Alas, my days of leisure in the UK are coming to an end. I leave here on February 1, returning in early May. By that time, the early camps will have been completed, and I will not be sorry to miss the summer heat and the exhausting humidity of the monsoon rains. Leaving Nepal was not as traumatic as I expected. The last ear camp in Rukum had been very busy, and the local people appreciated the work put in. At the end, there was little time to think, even less to go for meals with Nepali friends and families, as is usually the lovely but exhausting finale." Before her return to UK in May, after her next stint in Nepal, she would fit in five camps, the first starting the day after her arrival!

In her absence, Eka Dev and his team had run the Pokhara camps office well. He had communicated with the hospitals to be visited, arranged flights, and packed up all necessary equipment. The gynaecology camp was in Surkhet, a low-lying valley in the Inner Terai. One of the visiting anaesthetists, Neil Pollock from New Zealand, had worked short spells in Nepal previously. He wrote about the camp:

"Before leaving, official advice had been to avoid travel to Nepal, but people closer to the action said it was OK. The greatest risk was on the Nepali roads where traffic overtakes whenever the smallest gap appears, even on blind corners or hills. The 11-hour journey took us south, close to the Indian border and then back into the Himalayan foothills. It was not the most comfortable journey in the jeep, but the scenery was superb. Every piece of usable land was farmed.

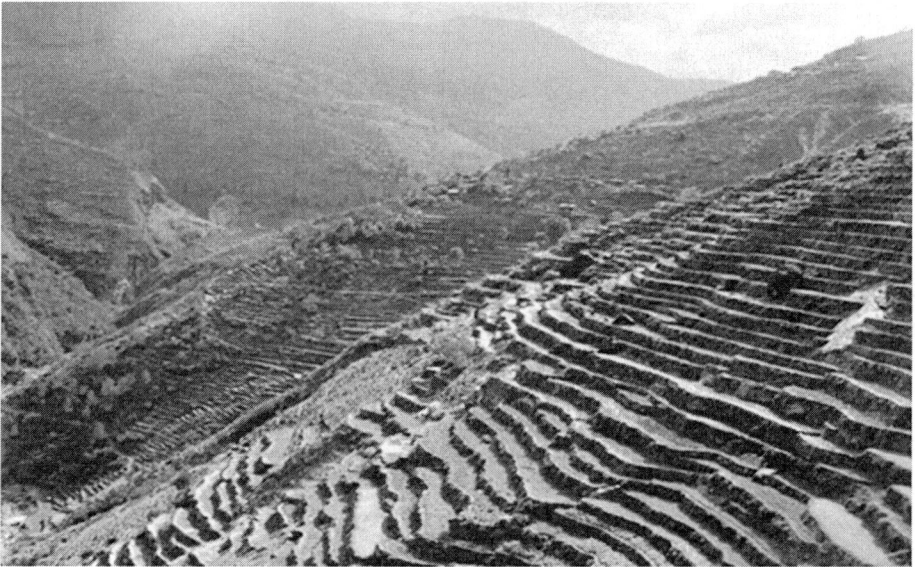

*Some typical terraced fields in the mid hills of Nepal. Farmers rotate crops of rice, maize, millet, wheat and other cereals according to season and altitude.*

"We travelled through numerous villages built on steep hillsides, with occasional dwellings on almost vertical slopes. News of the camp had been spread by radio and word of mouth. Some patients walked four or five days to get help. Language was no real problem as we had expat nurses and one gynaecologist who spoke Nepali well. A small hospital, with no proper surgical facilities, had been set up by the advance party, and we had one room and two 'operating tables', for two anaesthetists, two surgeons and two patients, side by side—a bit different from home! Between us, we did 15–16 vaginal hysterectomies a day, fitting in minor operations—a heavy workload!

"There were two major emergencies. One was a post-op patient who bled heavily. We had no ready source of blood, so we scavenged the blood in the abdomen, filtered it through sterile swabs and back into the patient—who survived.

"The second would also have been a critical case at home. A woman was noticed bundled up in blankets. She was very pregnant and had been carried six hours by her husband. She had had an eclamptic fit, very dangerous. A Caesarean Section was performed. The baby was dead, the mother deeply unconscious and

103

remained so for three days. Could we get a helicopter to take her to ICU in Kathmandu? No, was the answer. She had cerebral oedema and probably hypoxia. We used our powerful drugs, with little response. On the third day, Ellen had a feeling she would wake up and be hungry and bought some supplies. And amazingly, that was just what happened!"

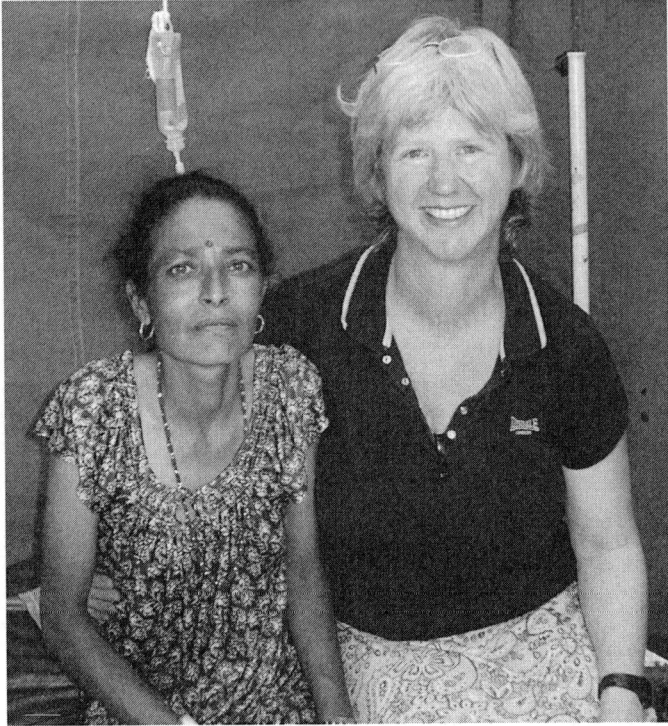

*Gynaecologist, Sarah Caukwell, with the lady who survived a massive haemorrhage.*

He also commented that many of the women had reduced lung function. The amount of oxygen in their bodies was nearer 90% than the usual 98%. This was probably due to smoking, but also because, in the home, wood fires and stoves burn in the centre of the room, creating much dust and smoke.

Of course, these dramatic events, and most camps have them, get the attention. Much quiet, undramatic work is done, mainly in the Outpatient Department, where minor issues are dealt with, reassurance is given, good screening takes place, and people requiring surgery are prepared.

All change for the next camp, a surgical one planned for nearby Ghorahi. It had been double-booked with the government family planning camp due to occur at the same time. There was no space available. At the last minute, the camp was swapped to Pyuthan. The team was gladly received and treated almost royally by the Medical Superintendent, Dr Ananda Shrestha. He provided sleeping places, lunch and an evening meal. Such luxury!

This was the first of ten annual surgical camps led by Ian Bissett. Having been challenged as a medical student in Auckland, New Zealand, by the inequalities of healthcare around the world, he spent his three-month elective period at Amppipal Hospital, set on a ridge with magnificent Himalayan views, four hours' walk from the nearest road. Dr Tom Hale, the surgeon there, taught Ian about a range of diseases rarely seen in developed countries. Ian went to Nepal thinking he was going to be a General Practitioner in rural New Zealand; he came back thinking the world needed another surgeon! It was a revelation: "Suddenly, I saw all that could be offered by surgery in this situation, where there was basically nothing."

After qualifying, he trained as a surgeon, including orthopaedics and neurosurgery. In 1987, he and his wife, Jo and their two small daughters joined INF in Pokhara, where he worked for 11 years at WRH, performing a vast range of sometimes very major surgery, improvising with minimal equipment, and training a succession of Nepali surgeons. In 1998, the family returned to Auckland for the children's education, and Ian specialised in colorectal surgery. His colleagues were sympathetic to his aim of visiting Nepal yearly to work in surgical camps, and many of them accompanied him, joining the team.

Ian Bissett's motivation could be summed up by two of his favourite quotes:

"Where your talents and the world's needs cross, there lies your vocation." (Aristotle).

"Whatever you did for the least of these brothers and sisters of mine, you did it for me." (Jesus).

The team in Pyuthan was smaller than usual—the plan had been to use staff from Ghorahi, but they could not transfer. However, unusually, the local nurses helped, and extra beds were supplied for post-op patients. A wide range of general surgery was carried out, but specialist problems like burn contractures, cleft lip and palate, were referred either to Pokhara, the camp providing funding, or maybe to a future plastic surgery camp in Pyuthan as there were 15 of these patients. The commonest problem in outpatients was abdominal pain and when stool tests showed worms and Giardia, patients were given medicine for these problems. 923 patients were seen and 63 operations performed in 6 days. It was busy.

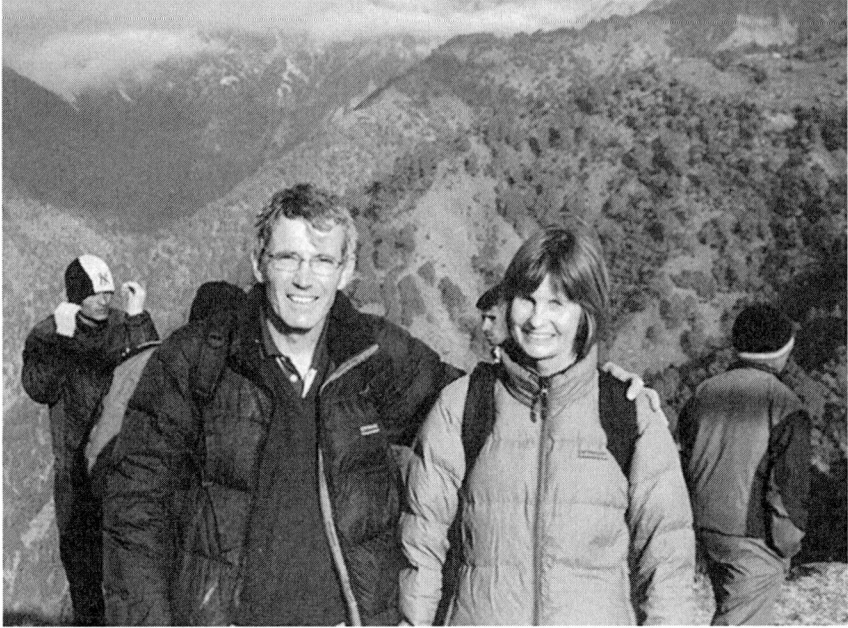

*Ian and his wife, Jo.*

Pyuthan lies in the middle of the Mahabharat range of hills, spreading right through the middle of Nepal and rising to 10,000 ft. Rivers cut through these hills. It is along these river valleys that paths and later, roads were built, on very unstable land. Most camps are held in these mountains and access is difficult. Pyuthan is the birthplace of Prachanda the founder of the Nepal Communist Party and leader of the Maoist revolts. Tensions were raised locally by the deaths of 12 Nepali workers in Iraq at the hands of ISIS (Islamic State). Mosques and Muslim shops were attacked all over Nepal. About 10% of Nepalis are Muslim, mainly in the south.

Tikapur, in the Far West region was the site for the next surgical camp. It is a town of 60,000, set on the banks of the Karnali River, a fine town with a wildlife park established by King Mahendra. Ellen's team had stayed previously in the national park. In April, this flat part of Nepal starts getting very hot, but whilst it is a long road journey, it is a good road. The only problem could be if the Maoists called a strike or closed the road.

The last gynaecology camp that year saw five women who, after difficult births, had developed a fistula. Fiona Burslam, a gynaecologist specialising in fistula repair, performed the complicated repair operations. She also assisted and taught Shirley Heywood, who commented, "It was great for me, but other members of the team were frustrated because of the time a complicated fistula repair takes and felt we should be concentrating on the women with prolapses, which could be huge and also desperately incapacitating". Camps are built around a rapid turnover, without taking risks. Post-op care of fistula patients takes a few weeks, keeping the bladder empty with a catheter whilst the wound heals. These five patients were transferred to Green Pastures in Pokhara for that care, and Fiona supervised it. All five had successful repairs. Another woman had a huge 10kg ovarian cyst removed. Some very satisfied and grateful women and families returned home.

It was very gratifying when a previous patient came to see the team at this camp. She had previously had huge fibroids preventing her from getting pregnant. She had visited other hospitals who recommended hysterectomy. But she wanted children. At an earlier gynaecology camp, a myomectomy was performed to remove the fibroids, and here she was, back with a lovely baby.

Shirley had a bad experience some years later, when two fistula repair patients in Surkhet did not receive proper post-op care and their catheters became blocked. The bladder filled and the wound burst. This had gone unnoticed because the night nurses were busy with maternity cases. Good nursing care was vital. In 2009, Shirley went to Ethiopia to enable her to become an expert in fistula care. After this camp, she realised that these repairs could not be done on camp, and they were referred to Patan Hospital in Kathmandu, or a new centre in Dharan in East Nepal.

After this final gynaecology camp was finished, Ellen rapidly packed her bags to meet her visa requirements, planning to return in October for the two final camps of that year.

# Chapter 14
## Demanding and Dangerous

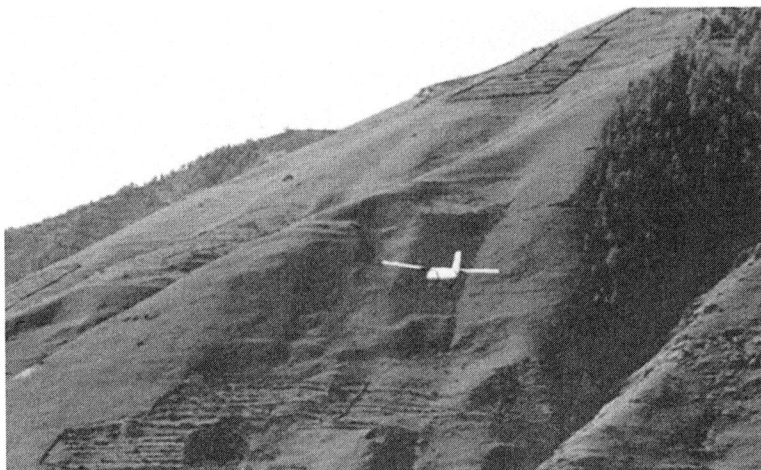

*A flight into the 'hills'.*

2005 was a difficult, demanding, dangerous year in Nepal. Few were unaffected by it. The Maoist insurgency was scenting victory, aiming at radical change which would see it at the heart of government. They carried the fight to the capital, blockading Kathmandu (which only had one real road into it), and bombs exploded in several areas, creating terror. Pokhara suffered similarly. The camps team had shifted one camp planned for Pokhara to elsewhere to avoid the danger. Local people in the Maoist-controlled area, which included most places where camps were held, told their stories. One woman came with her child, saying her husband had been forced to work on a road building gang. Another family had their house, land and livestock taken. Over 100,000 young men fled to India to avoid being drafted into the Maoist army. In February, King Gyanendra took back control from the government to deal with the insurgency. Fire fights between the rebels and the army and police increased, with many killed. Strikes were called and few broke them. Road blocks were set up. Advance notice (sometimes very short) was given for these.

The team continued to run medical camps in that environment, seeking to maintain morale in the hill towns and bring relief of suffering. Ellen's teams were courageous, wanting to press on wherever possible, helped by the fact that the Maoists had never caused the team any trouble. But the risk of being caught in crossfire was real. Patients also took great risks to get to the camps. Because of Maoist activity, two women, whose babies were breech presentations, could not get to the camp in time, and both babies died.

Ellen returned from the UK in February. The first camp, for gynaecology patients, went well. Despite the Maoist threat, 822 women were seen and 107 operations performed. No wonder they wanted to keep the camps going. As they travelled to the camp, they found the main road blocked. Taking the rough branch road, they came face to face with a Maoist Commander. His face was hard, but he allowed the team through, warning them that the road was about to be repaired and would be shut for six months. It was a long, hard 50 miles. Ellen takes up the story of the journey back from Arghakhanchi:

"We were uncertain how things would be. People warned us not to go by road but to go by helicopter. We heard weird and wonderful stories of roadblocks and bombs. I had peace of mind about going by road and the team were very laidback about the whole thing. After travelling a short time, we came to a landslide. Digging our way out was getting us nowhere. We could only pray, and then, after 20 minutes, suddenly, round a corner came a big JCB digger with a huge bucket on the front! It quickly cleared the landslide. We then drove south for four hours to the East-West Highway, stopping for rice to consider again what to do. There was no traffic. The road had been deserted for two days. We decided to go for it. Security forces were protecting the road and phoned ahead to say we were coming, and with empty roads, we were able to speed along 60 miles, then turn off onto the spur joining the Pokhara-Kathmandu road. Eventually we met a convoy of 175 buses and lorries accompanied by an armoured vehicle escort. Two convoys passed us going the other way. The amazing thing is that if we had waited another day at camp, the roads would have been blocked and we would still be there. A week after we left, the Maoists attacked the police post in Arghakhanchi. 40 Maoists and an unspecified number of police were killed and many injured. Offices in the town were bombed, as was the hospital admin block."

Three weeks later, they were due in Ghorahi for another gynaecology camp. The situation had deteriorated. An ambulance returning from taking a patient to

Nepalganj brought some people back. It was stopped and torched, but the people escaped. Small traders were being prevented from taking and selling their milk and vegetables, resulting in hardship. Ellen cancelled the trip to Ghorahi.

The next camp was a dental camp in Beni. Effective dental services are limited in the developing world, sometimes being provided by untrained practitioners in the bazaars, but the need is great. Particularly for young people, preventative dental work saves so much trouble later. The basic public health message of brushing teeth was being taught to those young people attending school. In the villages, whilst some things were improving, many young girls were still not receiving any education. Women do most of the agricultural and house work, as well as carrying water and firewood. Children with disability, including deafness, frequently missed out on school. Vaccinations, early treatment and good maternal health were all preventative measures that were lacking.

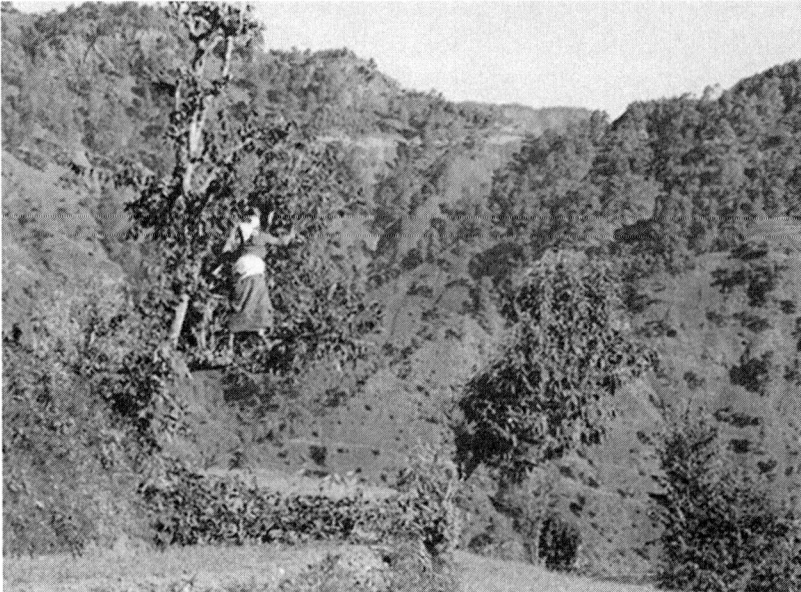

*A woman climbs a tree to cut winter fodder for her goats. Falls from trees are a major cause of trauma in Nepal.*

The April ear camp was scheduled for Beni, 12 years after the first one had been held there in 1993. There were difficulties. A general strike was due to take place during the camp. That created a problem for those travelling from abroad who had booked air tickets and hotels. The decision was made to switch to

Pyuthan, so an advance party was sent on ahead to set up the outpatients, audiology, theatre and pharmacy. The senior doctor in Pyuthan, Ananda Shrestha, was always glad to accommodate us at short notice. Mike Smith arrived with his colleagues. Two helicopters were required for the 10 people plus baggage and equipment. They landed in the school sports field and were greeted by large crowds of students.

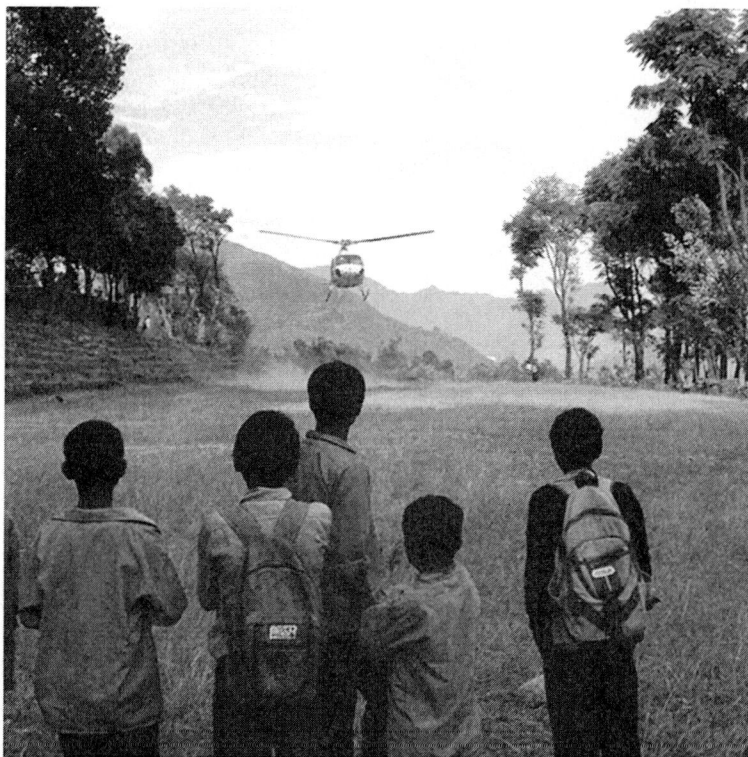

*Some of the schoolchildren gathered to see the arrival of the helicopter outside their school.*

The last camp before the monsoon was for plastic surgery in Musikot, precariously perched in the remote, high Himal, close to where the winter snowline reaches, a town full of small, dark, smoky houses. At previous camps in Rukum, there had been several patients requiring plastic surgery. During this camp, it became obvious that there were many other surgical needs. Two surgeons were present with two anaesthetists. One of the surgeons, Dr Richard Schwartz, was the medical superintendent at Green Pastures Hospital, responsible for rehabilitation and leprosy surgery. The initial turnout was poor.

Confusing messages had been given on the radio and letters sent had not arrived. Not surprising in the midst of national upheaval.

The decision had been made to fly in. Ellen wrote home with a graphic description of the flight: "We went to Rukum on the 'vomit comet'! That is the only way I can describe the flight from Pokhara to Rukum. Whilst some of us were going greener and greener, others were filling plastic bags. Before going, I felt God say, 'I will send an angel before you.' As the plane went up and down, then from side to side—the wings too close to the hills for my liking—I kept reassuring myself with that promise. When we eventually landed, feeling very shaky, the pilot said, 'I thought we were not going to make it.'"

After a slow start, all manner of pathologies presented themselves. Patients from previous camps called in to say all was well. Several cleft palates and hare lips were repaired. Poorly healed scars and contractures resulting from burns were the most common presentation. A number of general surgical operations were also performed. Where possible, patients were given appropriate treatment, including one man who was not a patient, but Ellen noticed that he looked dreadful. He was very anaemic, though it was not clear why. Two of the team gave a unit of blood for him, and he was a new man the next day. Following surgery, several children were referred to Pokhara for speech therapy and needed help with their costs. The hospital doctor and staff looked after the 58 patients who had operations. It was good to see a well-staffed medical service in such a remote place. There was no mention made of the return journey in the team's records, but obviously they made it!

# Chapter 15

## Vital Contributors

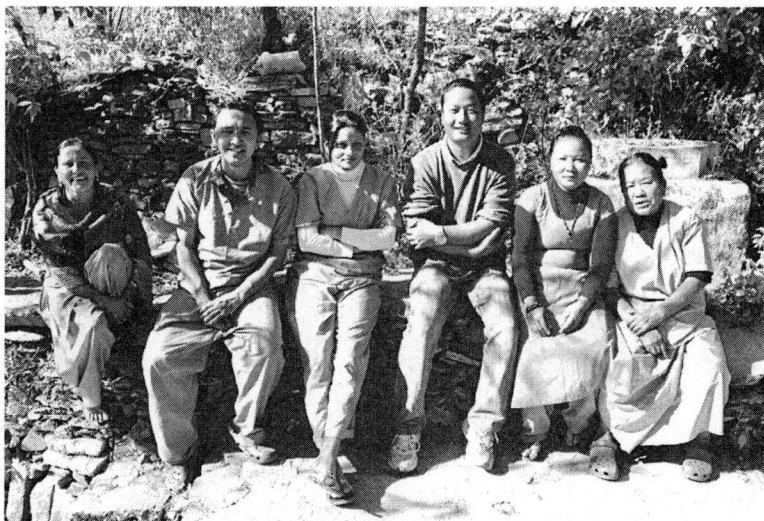

*Just a few of the regular team: Anandi, Robin, Dil Kumari, Rabi Gurung, Indra and Regina.*

Whilst the most prominent members of the team were the surgeons, they would be unable to work without a substantial support team. The essential equipment had to be prepared. Team members such as Rabi Gurung, who was the technician for many years, were a great asset. Rabi was responsible for checking technical equipment such as operating microscopes and audiometers, which had to be carefully cleaned and stored, and surgical instruments checked for damage. Rabi was incredibly resourceful and always had a smile and can-do attitude. He would repair the generator, string up the electrics and lights, tenderly carry a child out from the operating room to its mother, then turn around and fix an autoclave.

Expensive equipment can be destroyed by fungus and damp in the monsoon, when humidity is often 100%—one of many good reasons for not holding camps in the monsoon season. Items were stored between camps in 'hot boxes', metal cabinets and tin trunks with a light bulb inside to keep the items warm and reduce humidity and a bag of silica gel to absorb moisture.

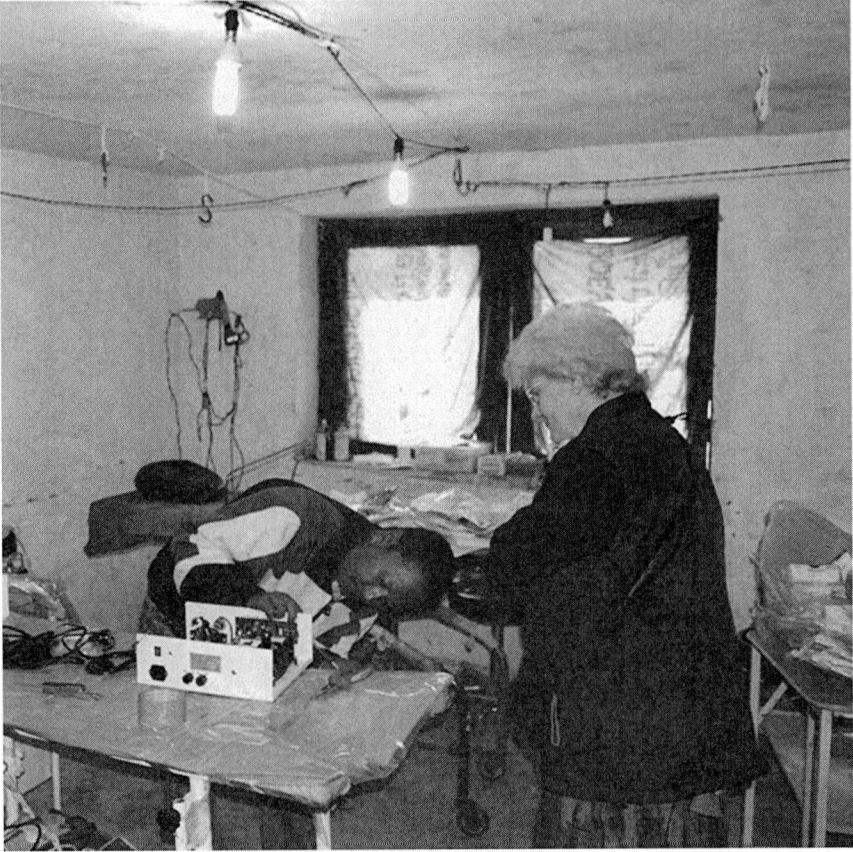

*Ellen and Rabi Gurung: Essential maintenance.*

At the end of a camp large blue plastic drums came back to Pokhara full of wet, dirty linen. All these had to be packed up, taken back to base, cleaned, dried, sterilised and repackaged for the next camp. Gauze squares used during surgery, and as dressings, were cut from muslin sheets and carefully folded up by the ladies in the team. Wooden sticks with soft cotton wool were used to mop out pus from ears, enabling the eardrums to be seen and a diagnosis made. These were prepared from large sections of bamboo, sliced and carved down to exact sizes. Sometimes there were only 10 days between camps and the Nepali team could be rushed off their feet with so much work.

The vehicles, a truck, elderly Land Rovers, and a Tata jeep, had to be cleaned and maintained. They were frequently used on rough roads, and breakdowns could present a nightmare scenario. The drivers needed skill to be safe on Nepali roads, where corners are routinely cut by buses and unstable lorries, often travelling too fast. Road maintenance is poor.

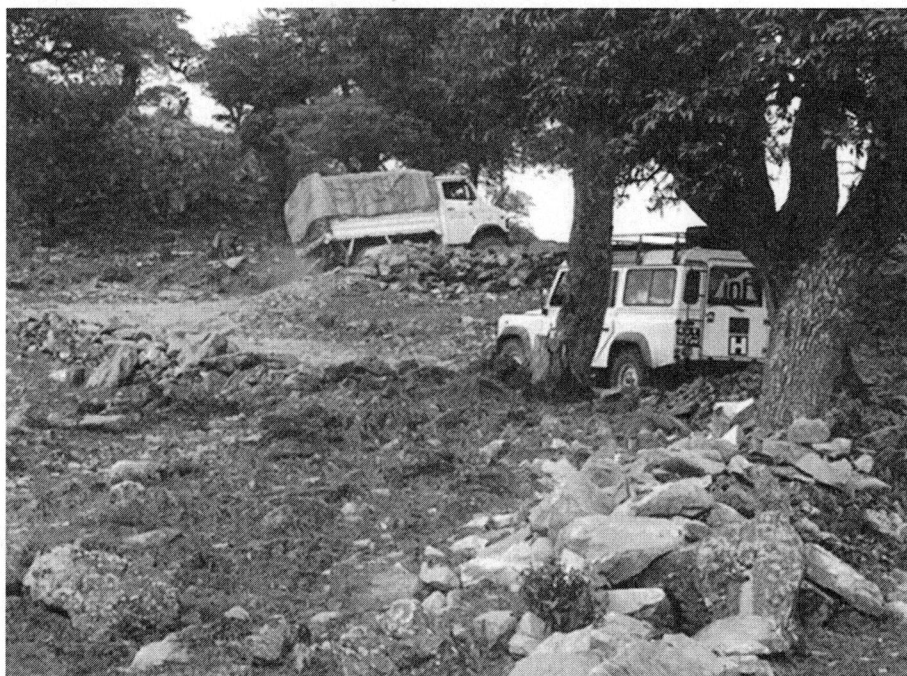

*The INF vehicles and drivers cope with another tough road.*

Fortunately, camps rarely operated in the monsoons when landslides are common, but it is always possible to meet a boulder in the road. In the dry season, some roads are dust bowls. On the road trip to remote Accham in the Far West region in 2006, one Land Rover broke down en-route and it, with its cargo of people and baggage, had to be towed by the other, on to the next town. Repair could involve an overnight stay in "an absolutely dirty hotel." Happy days! When a vehicle broke down, even after a long period behind the wheel, drivers like Prithvi Raj and Min Gurung would immediately be underneath the bonnet or on the ground under the vehicle, identifying the problem and working out a solution. On one journey, they got stuck in the mud once and the dust twice, on deeply rutted tracks. "Everyone rose to the occasion, putting vehicle mats, stones, weeds and tree branches on the road to give the vehicles some grip." Punctures were common, and when more than one wheel is affected, miles from any help, vehicles have to shuttle to get assistance. On one trip, the brakes of one Land Rover were constantly overheating, necessitating frequent stops to pour precious drinking water on the discs. Alarming on the steep, narrow roads! More than once a shock absorber or spring broke but local ingenuity often resolved the problem.

The drivers in the team were amazing, often somehow remaining alert and awake for many hours, then, on the camp, doing other work such as patient registrations, fetching and carrying. This willingness to do more menial tasks was a hallmark of all the team members, an attitude which is not normal in the rigid caste system. However, the team could see the service being delivered to the people and the readiness of visiting professionals to carry boxes or push vehicles and this seemed to rub off. They were rightly proud of their work.

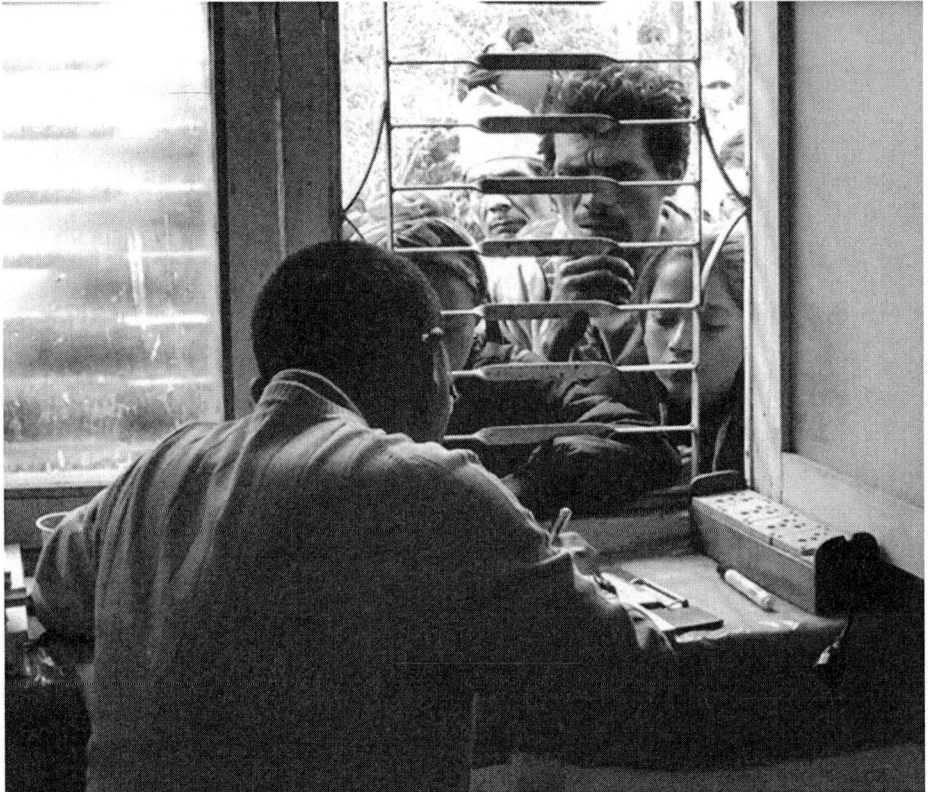

*Staff often worked flexibly, taking on roles such as patient registration.*

Robin Lama was a very good scrub nurse and fulfilled a vital role. Ellen's concern for him was that he had no formal training, which he would need if he was eventually to work in government service. Helping team members to get recognised qualifications and training became an increasing responsibility.

Anaesthetists were a vital, if not always seen, part of the medical team. For one of the 2005 camps, the booked anaesthetist had to return to Australia because of family illness. Ellen was in Kathmandu, and it just happened that she bumped into a visitor who was an anaesthetist, Maurice Lee, who agreed to come on camp. Hysterectomies could be performed under spinal anaesthetic, which surgeons can learn. They can also deal with more minor problems using local anaesthetic. Major ear surgery in higher income countries is mainly done under general anaesthetic. However, because of a lack of anaesthetists at early camps, Mike started doing operations with local anaesthetic and sedation. The tough local people tolerated this surprisingly well, even many children. This, however, was not ideal and once there were regular anaesthetists such as Charlie Collins and David Hill, they greatly improved the techniques. General anaesthetic with only basic facilities, especially for surgery on the head, was difficult, as the surgeon and the anaesthetist were competing for space. The availability of Ketamine made such a difference, increasing the safety margins. The painful local anaesthetic ear block could be put in with the patient already anaesthetised by an injection of Ketamine. The anaesthetist straight out from home needed to rapidly rethink the technique needed in an isolated place with no cylinder gases and, supremely, no oxygen. Sometimes the team carried a device called an oxygen concentrator, but it was bulky and heavy and at altitude it is hard to know whether it is producing much additional oxygen. Learning to work with local facilities was also new for most surgeons used to a Western medical environment. The patient might move, which for delicate middle ear surgery can be challenging!

The cleaners and helpers were another vital part of the team. They worked late at night, hand washing surgical drapes and instruments, then repacking and sterilising them in large pressure cookers. These were usually heated by Primus-style kerosene stoves but, on at least one camp, over wood fires. Often, during the day, the drapes were to be seen laid over bushes drying in the sun so that the ultraviolet rays helped to kill germs.

Sometimes, local Nepalis, such as hotel owners, played an important role: "Although our hotels left a lot to be desired, the owner of the one in Achham went out of his way to help. Maurice Coutanceau (anaesthetist) had put his suitcase on the table to be collected the next morning, not realising that the table doubled up as bed for one of the hotel workers. When we got to the bottom of the long hill, we were waved down 'There is a case left in the hotel.' No phones, but the messages were shouted from hill to hill! The hotel owner came after us in a jeep and delivered the case to Maurice as he was getting on the plane. Timing was perfect!!"

The visitors all had to fly into Kathmandu. From Europe, that always meant an overnight flight, with at least one change, in the Gulf, Istanbul or Delhi. It is possible to fly home westwards with the sun in one long day. From Australia, the change would usually be in Singapore, Bangkok or maybe Hong Kong. This meant arriving tired and jetlagged and required at least one night in Kathmandu to recover before travelling on, by plane or road, to camp—exciting, of course, for the newcomer but wearing and with inevitable culture shock. Nepal previously had its own international airline (Royal Nepal Airlines Corporation, RNAC, sometimes known to foreigners as Really Nothing Absolutely Certain!). It used to be possible to fly from Kathmandu to Frankfurt and London with them but not now. Following trouble with one plane, probably an electrical fault, two goats were sacrificed in front of it to the sky god.

It is not only in Nepal that travel can be difficult. Ellen's flight out of Glasgow en route to Nepal was only confirmed four hours before departure. Mike and team had an emergency landing in Azerbaijan, when there was a fire in the hold; long delays in Delhi with storms; and two overnight stops, each when a wheel on the plane wouldn't work, once in Kathmandu and once in Heathrow!

A ceasefire was agreed in Nepal after the monsoon. The next three camps took place at this beautiful time of year when the rice ripens and is harvested— a busy time when usually less patients come to the hospitals, as everyone is reaping, winnowing and storing or selling the rice. It is also the time of the two major festivals: Dashain (which lasts 10 days and for which many people travel back to their families) and Diwali (known as Tihar in Nepal), the Festival of Lights. Nevertheless, the three camps, one each of gynaecology, ear and surgery, saw 1,874 people come for help, with 307 requiring operations.

At surgical camps, a general practitioner helped screen patients for the surgeons to see, and at one surgical camp, in Arghakhanchi, a radiographer was present to perform 142 ultrasounds during the seven-day camp. Most of the surgical cases had one of several different types of hernia repaired, 17 patients had gallbladder removal, but two with kidney stones proved very difficult. A few were referred to a regional centre at camp's expense. Money was also provided for an older man who had a kidney stone removed with difficulty, to pay someone else to do his work while he recovered. This was a very cold camp, and many of the team caught coughs and colds. Ellen had wondered why someone had sent her three packs of 'Fisherman's Friends' (a throat lozenge). Now she knew! Camp finished on December 6, and Ellen was on her way home on

December 8, leaving the team to clear up. No rush there, then!

At the beginning of 2006 the cease-fire ended. Lack of agreement between government and rebels opened the door for a final push by the rebels. This was to create problems for the team. There was plenty to test Ellen's faith! The first camp was to be in Surkhet, but she was unwilling to subject the team of 21 members to the long two-day road journey, when strikes and roadblocks were increasingly common. Someone asked: "When will you come to Beni for a gynaecology camp?" As is clear, Ellen's heart was always for the poor and, particularly, for the women, whose lot in life was very hard in a male-dominated society. To Beni they went.

"We were inundated with patients. Our two GPs examined 800 women, whilst our two surgeons with one anaesthetist, plus an assistant, coped with 113 operations. Fortunately, they were all very hard working. Our focus, as always, was on the well-being of our patients. Again, we had to be 'listening ears' to many women full of anxiety—some whose husbands had been killed by the Maoists, others who had had abortions and couldn't cope with the loss of the baby. Another, unable to have children, was terrified to tell her family. 'They will throw me out. Society will despise me.' She wept and wept. Later, she allowed us to tell her father. One woman had sold her land and spent a year's wages on radiotherapy. Now she needed a hysterectomy but had no money and could not borrow any. Surgery was performed and happily, there was no sign of cancer spreading.

"Just as camp was finishing, a nationwide strike was called. Our doctors needed to catch an international flight. What to do? We decided to drive. Two hours later, we reached a road blocked by trees and with a pressure cooker bomb visible. We decided to stay the night and were guided to a nice hotel by a former paramedic with whom Ellen had worked. The next day was decision time – to call for a (very expensive) helicopter to get our doctors and others out for their flight or to try the road. I felt: try the road. We parked up beside the block, walked over it and found a car on the other side to take us to Pokhara for them to fly to Kathmandu."

The next camp was for ears in Bajura, rated 74th out of 75 districts in Nepal in the poverty stakes. Mugu next door was ranked 75th. Because the walk from the nearest airport was an eight-hour stretch, the decision had been made to go by helicopter.

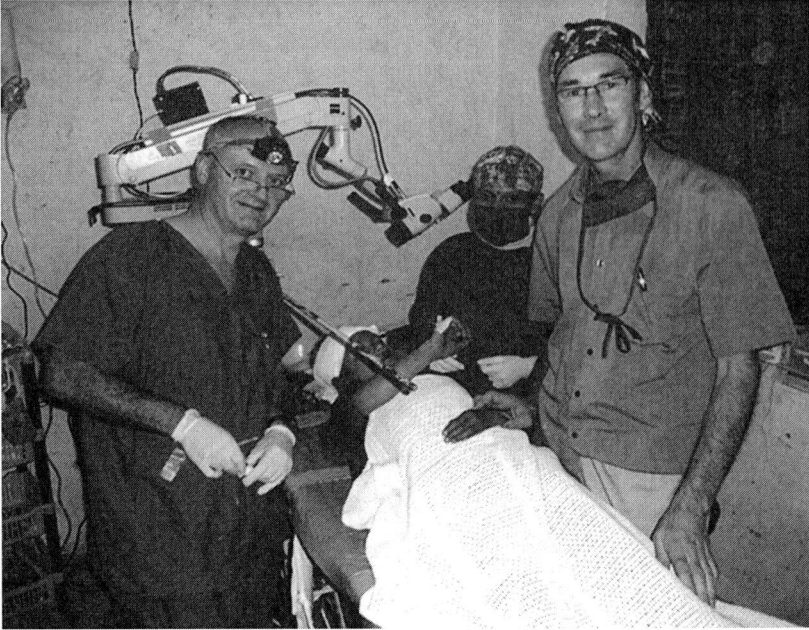

*Alan Bennett, anaesthetist from the UK with Wayne Butt, ENT surgeon from NZ, in Bajura. Both joined many camps, sometimes at very short notice, to fill unexpected gaps.*

Again, for Ellen, this was a step of faith as there was not enough money in the kitty. Opening her emails, she found further promises of money. It was paid for. The way money was given and arrived at the right time is a constant source of wonderment.

"The poverty was extreme. Food was only adequate for six months of the year. Clothing was in tatters, and it was bitterly cold here in the mountains. In many areas, women wear their wealth in gold earrings or nose piercings. There was no sign of that here. But it was lovely to hear the patients saying, 'No others are doing what you people are doing.' 'You operate on us, give us food and clothing. What kind of people are you?'

"Because it was busy here, with 824 outpatients and 124 operations, we decided to stay and work an extra day. Just as well, as the rain poured down and clouds covering the mountains would have made it impossible for the helicopter." Winter rains are unusual, and the snowline can drop below 9,000 ft. It was even colder! They had many requests to return for a gynaecology camp.

The drama was not quite over for those trying to get back to Kathmandu for flights. When they arrived at Nepalganj airport, now in hot weather, there were no taxis waiting—another strike! Eventually, two taxis turned up and took the team to a hotel and a welcome hot shower—luxury after Bajura.

There was a further ear camp in Beni before Ellen returned home, but camps were now able to run even in her absence.

As Mike was walking on the path between wards in Beni a young man called him. "I was your patient at the Western Regional Hospital about 10 years ago". He opened his shirt to show scars. When this man was only 10 years old he had accidentally swallowed alkali (lye) that was stored in an old juice bottle and was used for making soap. His whole gullet (oesophagus) from top to bottom had become so scarred and narrow that he was unable to eat, and had become very thin and malnourished, barely surviving. After some weeks of building him up with high calories and protein delivered by a tube directly into his stomach, Ian Bissett and Mike had operated, to bring a section of the boy's large intestine up through his chest, and join it between his stomach and throat, to replace his damaged oesophagus. Neither Ian nor Mike had even seen this done before, but amazingly, the very day of the planned surgery, a thoracic surgeon from the USA visited the hospital and was able to assist them. When Mike asked, in the Beni camp, if all was well, the young man said, "Yes, I am absolutely fine, apart from a bit of heartburn!" They subsequently did a similar procedure for two or three other patients. One of these had taken a drink from what he thought was a beer bottle but it contained acid for work in the small village goldsmith shop.

Rather bravely, towards the end of the monsoon, in stifling heat and humidity, a dental camp was arranged for Taulihawa, a town of 27,000 people right on the border with Uttar Pradesh in northern India. This is a great area for Buddhist pilgrimage; Siddhartha Gautama, known as the Buddha, was born nearby in 563BC. A small team of six people attended the dental camp with Hilary Dell Cook as the dentist, Robin Lama (the usual assistant), the driver doubling as registrar, two crowd controllers and Eka Dev. The facilities they were offered at the hospital initially were totally inadequate, with no electricity, no water and no fan! The doctor was absent, only arriving at the end. A better room was provided by a helpful nurse.

On the first of the six days, only 25 patients came, typical of slow starts in new areas. There was only one dentist. 309 patients were seen and 200 turned away! There were 186 fillings done, 132 extractions and 50 scalings. Seven patients were referred on to bigger hospitals. The workload was heroic in the fierce heat. Following this, a plastic surgery camp was carried out in WRH, Pokhara, where patients referred from other camps came for their surgery for cleft palates. The warm weather made these procedures safer in small children. The surgical team came from Alder Hey Children's Hospital, Liverpool. Rosie Sleator, an INF speech therapist working in Pokhara, was present to organise their follow up. Rosie, from Northern Ireland was immensely popular and is still remembered many years later by her patients.

# Chapter 16

## To Earth's Remotest End

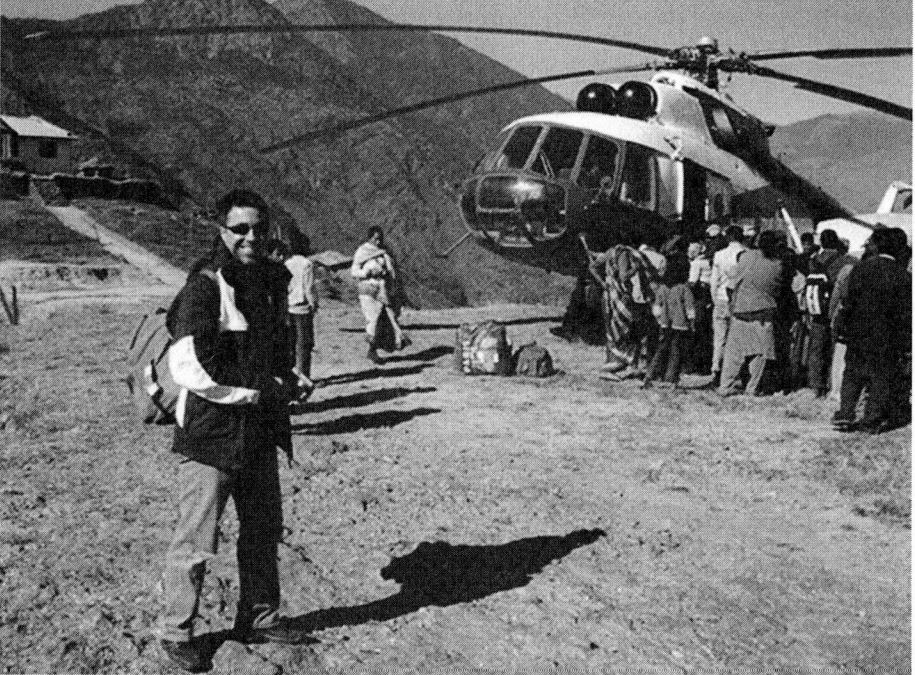

*Dr Lukas Eberle waiting for the helicopter, Kalikot.*

The traveller, flying from Delhi across the flat Ganges plain to Kathmandu, sees what appears to be clouds on the horizon. He gradually realises that these are, in fact, the snows of the Himalayas. Suddenly the land folds into a long line of hills, tree-clad ridges and snowy peaks. The Indian and Asian tectonic plates collide, forcing upwards the youngest and greatest mountain ranges on the planet. The Himalayas are still growing at the rate of about 6 cm per year, much of which is lost to erosion and the mountains collapsing under their own weight. Earth tremors and occasional earthquakes contribute to the instability of the terrain, increasing the already frequent landslides.

It was to this land that INF came to work, in 1952. Having established the Shining Hospital and Green Pastures in the Pokhara valley, the mission gradually began to branch out westwards. In the late 1970s, the Nepali government invited INF to head up a TB/Leprosy programme throughout the western part of Nepal. Later, community development projects began in the remotest and neediest areas.

Ellen returned from home leave in 2006 to a peaceful Nepal. The Maoists, seeing their aim being fulfilled, joined the government and parliament. The need for change was clear. Hopefully, with a peace (which will take time to work through), roads can be built, education improved, especially in the smaller communities, and hospitals can be equipped and staffed. The aim of the Maoists was an end to the feudal system, dating back over 200 years. After much discussion, the government sought to put the country back on its feet.

The camps team was attempting to get to areas that had previously been closed to outside personnel—usually because of political unrest. The three winter camps were far-flung and difficult to access. It would be a first visit to Achham, remote, in the far west, near Bajura. The dreadful journey to get there, with breakdowns, delays, and bedbugs, has already been mentioned. "This was a combined dental and ear camp. The dental camp, planned late on, had not been properly advertised. Nevertheless, 91 people were seen, and the fact that there were 126 extractions and only 24 fillings showed how poor the care for teeth was in this place. A man came with a large tumour in the roof of his mouth, too risky to remove on a camp. The team explained and hoped he would travel to Pokhara, where they could arrange surgery.

The ear camp was quieter than most. Mike Smith and team were back. Ellen gave reasons for smaller numbers. "These people have a hand-to-mouth existence. Hardship and hunger are a way of life." There were some lovely responses. "We have never had help like this before. No one comes here." The Maoist district commander was again encouraging. "You people are very welcome. This is the type of service we want in the remote areas. No harm will come to you." They worked late on the last night. A man rushed in at 5 pm when the operating lists were full. He had mistaken the date and had, as his feet testified, walked five days. He had his operation. Ellen wanted to get Tee shirts printed, "I survived Achham"!

At the end of November, a revisit to Achham was planned but it was transferred to another remote area, Rolpa, on the slopes of the Dhaulagiri mountain range. This time, it was a general surgical camp, led by Ian Bissett, accompanied by his colleagues from New Zealand. One man had come to Libang, the main town in Rolpa, with his wife, to get citizenship papers. "Do you remove abdominal lumps? My wife has had one for 10 years." So as an incidental to the man's visit, Ian removed a 6lb cyst from her abdomen! A 10-year-old boy was found, by ultrasound, to have stones in both kidneys. After a difficult experience at an earlier camp, Ian decided this was not appropriate for him to do here. The camp decided to pay all the costs to send him to Kathmandu for his surgery. Subsequently, we heard that they had made the long journey. All went well and he returned, healthy, to Rolpa. Five years previously, his father had gone to work in the Gulf and had not been heard of since.

The team was given a warm welcome in Rolpa and was invited to return. Sandra Chinnery was there; she loved being part of the team and worked with Ellen for many years. She commented: "The main town is Libang. The hospital is conveniently (!) situated an hour from the town in splendid isolation. Breakfast was deep fried bread and fried batter 'jeli' rings soaked in syrup. It took two days to fully prepare the room to make it fit for surgery; there were more patients than beds, so patients lay on concrete floors and many chose to be out in the sun whilst recovering. It was cold!"

The team had planned to go to Bajura again. They got as far as Surkhet, where they were supposed to catch the helicopter. Then the helicopter broke down and would take a month to repair! "Thank goodness we had not got to Bajura. It would have taken us two days to walk out, and what about the equipment, and flights back to Europe! So another change of plan: Let's see if we can stay in Surkhet. One of the Surkhet medical officers had been negative towards camps in the past, but he had left for a fortnight's leave two days before we arrived. Perfect! A very good camp was held there." He was probably concerned that he would be left with the responsibility of dealing with any complications and had little knowledge of the specialty. The team always went to great lengths to avoid this.

Small wonder then, that Ellen wrote afterwards to supporters: "Remember the teams in these remote locations. Pray for good team spirit; for the wellbeing of patients, for the skills of surgeons and anaesthetists, for stamina to work long hours, for good health, for the ability to cope with the deprivations of remote living, for the logistics of moving 21 people around the country."

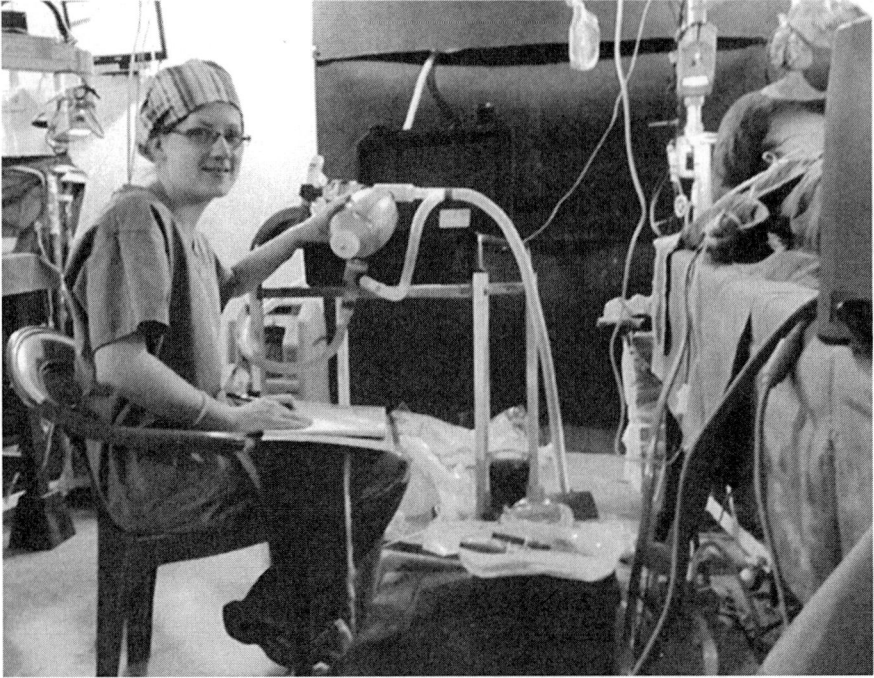

*Becky Paris was brought up in Nepal when her parents worked there. After qualifying as an anaesthetist she returned to help camps and other medical projects. Here she is using a simple portable device to provide general anaesthesia.*

At this point, Ellen resigned from INF, after 35 years, though she continued to work with them. The new visa situation only allowed her to work for five months each year. Her church had a ruling that, unless a person worked six months a year abroad, it could not continue to give support. She felt morally she could not go on receiving money from people in her church. "Nevertheless, I will continue to have input into camps until a replacement appears."

Camps did not stop because Ellen's visa restricted her time in Nepal. A strategically different gynaecology camp was held in early January in Surkhet. This was carefully planned and took place in the transformed, newly opened Mid-West Regional Hospital. The Medical Superintendent was actively involved, and the hospital nurses cared for the post-op patients. In addition, it was used as a doctors' training camp. Two doctors came from Jumla and one trainee gynaecologist in Surkhet, to add to their skills, and the resident gynaecologist was also fully involved. INF had worked for years in different health projects in this area, and in the next decade, they built a facility for inpatient beds for leprosy treatment and rehabilitation, known as the Shining Hospital Surkhet. Shirley Heywood was now an INF visa-holding gynaecologist

126

there. The British Government Department for International Development (DFID) were funding the care of patients. Prior to the camp, local health posts had been visited and all patients had already been screened, so there were not the usual vast numbers of outpatients.

The majority of women had a prolapsed uterus, some the size of a football, and were treated by vaginal hysterectomy with repair. A few had abdominal hysterectomy, including one with a hydatidiform mole, presenting as a 26-week size pregnancy. She was later given Methotrexate as a protection against it being cancerous. Only one had a fistula, following a difficult birth. She had had incontinence for 30 years, having lost that baby and 15 others. At last, she could get help. 75 operations were performed and much teaching took place. For some, camp had to end two days early. A strike had been called, so part of the team left, returning to Kathmandu for their international flights.

Shirley Heywood wrote a glowing report afterwards: "I had been out to several health posts, including one a four-hour Land Rover journey away. Some women had walked two days to get to the health post and were given dates to come to Surkhet for surgery. It was particularly satisfying that the Nepali MD gynaecologist operated on more patients than he ever had before. The paramedic anaesthetist from Jumla had always looked frightened if I did surgery in Jumla. Now he worked with experienced anaesthetists and his confidence grew—vital for Jumla. Surkhet's laboratory technician also learned a great deal. The visitors from New Zealand rapidly adjusted to equipment they had never used before and many shortages. The theatre staff from both hospitals learned a lot from the very experienced Nepali nurse, Regina." Eka Dev, the co-ordinator said "It was a wonderful camp."

Shirley touched on the visa problem: "Prior to the camp, I was concerned that I had not yet renewed my registration as a doctor in Nepal. Every year, a new application has to be made. My passport, with those of other INFers, was in a ministry office in Kathmandu whilst the new government sorted out what to do about my visa, what to charge. The visa is needed prior to registration. This is a slow process (it also means you cannot leave the country). On Jan 1st, the Nepal Medical Council had one topic—what to do about re-registering INF doctors. They agreed to accept provisional letters from the visa ministry, so my registration was done just in time." She also sketched out the political situation: "Whilst the cease-fire held, there was an increase in unrelated violence. The Nepali Parliament had seven parties, and the Maoists were to become the eighth.

127

Elections were planned for later. There were, unsurprisingly, various opposing forces, and the country needed a new constitution."

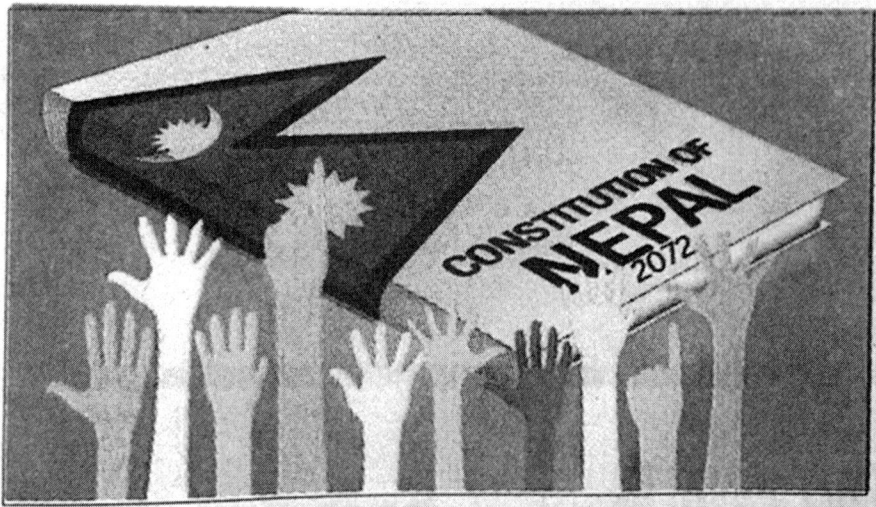

*As in this newspaper article, hopes were high for a new constitution and federal structure, but it was delayed several years.*

The next camp was a dental camp in Jumla. Good luck to anybody going to Jumla in mid-winter with the resin from burning pinewood coating everything, and the cold. How on earth dentists can keep their fingers working is hard to imagine. But the patients were very grateful, and Jumla was soon to change for the better.

Sometimes, it seemed that life in the hills had been better with the Maoists in control. Now, it seemed, any group with a grievance could block roads or declare a strike. The police had become so decimated they did not want to get involved. The gynaecology camp in Rolpa was hampered by several problems delaying travel, but Shirley Heywood and her team met many needs.

Mike and his team of ear surgeons flew from the UK and on to Nepalganj. That flight was horrendous, hitting a storm that caused the plane to drop 500 ft and threw them around. The pilot could not continue the flight and had to return to Kathmandu, where they stayed overnight. Poor weather delayed the flight next morning. Having arrived at 11 am, they then had a 16-hour Land Rover journey on the twisting, ascending and descending road to Doti District in the Far West Region, with snow on the side of the road. Arriving at 3 am, the team collapsed into their sleeping bags.

Sarah Puttix (nee Scott Brown) wrote about the road journey: "The first few hours were along the E-W highway in the Terai. It was straight and flat on a raised dike, between miles of emerald green rice fields, wattle and daub villages, jungle, where we saw monkeys, peacocks and deer and even some crocodiles (Gharial), in one of the rivers we crossed. It was very beautiful and different from the hills and hill villages. Many of the houses made the leaning tower of Pisa look stable, and there were whole villages of plastic sacks stretched over sticks, with a few skinny goats, and lots of skinny children. The next six or more hours were spent winding up into the hills through rhododendron forests, just coming into flower; tiny houses built along the road, with the backs of the houses perched over the edge of precipitous drops and rice fields carved out of unfeasibly steep slopes.

"My anaesthetist colleague knew some Nepali language. The Nepali staff thought it was hilarious that when he swatted a fly (makha), he would say he had killed a fish (machha). It took three days, and scores of flies before they put him right! The scrubbed surgeons and patients tolerated the thwacks of the fly swat well, mid operation. On another occasion an anaesthetist kept using the phrase 'lamo lamo las phernos', to patients he was preparing for surgery, (meaning to say, 'lamo lamo sas phernos'). Instead of encouraging deep breaths, he was suggesting a change of a very long corpse!"

Rooms in the simple district hospital had been provided, but the usual team cleaning took some hours. They had room for three operating tables. They had three surgeons but only two anaesthetists, who were going to be kept busy! Mike Carter, one of the anaesthetists, wrote: "One room became the operating theatre, with three operating tables, each with a microscope, two with TV screens for teaching. There was just enough space for the surgeons, and Sarah and I to move between and care for patients. We only gave two full general anaesthetics, to the two youngest (3-year olds) having major surgery, and we gave ketamine sedation to the under-twelves. When a patient was ready for the surgeon, a walkie-talkie summoned them from out-patients, 100 metres away. It was a first-class service in third world conditions. Imagine a patient walking from north of the Himalayas for four days to reach us. The surgeon and audiologist see her on the day she arrives at 5pm. Within an hour she has her operation! (Mike Smith recognised the referral note she brought with her, as from a doctor he had trained years before!)"

At first, patients were slow to come, as it was very cold and wet, but warmer days saw the crowds arriving. As always, Mike was willing to work into the late evening if there were patients waiting for surgery. Even in the most diseased ears, he always tried to reconstruct the hearing apparatus, often reshaping and fitting the small hearing bones, or using tiny bone grafts (ossiculoplasty), to replace those eroded by infection. His teams worked very hard! It was good that the Regional Director of Health for the Far Western Region and the local Chief District Officer (CDO) visited this camp and saw the work. The director had asked the team to come.

This camp provided free treatment to all. Until now, deposits had been paid by surgical patients to make sure they turned up. Many patients were seen: 915 in outpatients, 319 for audiograms with 93 hearing aids fitted—always a very busy department—203 ears were syringed, and 101 operations performed, most of them major. As usual, a range of other patients arrived and were treated if possible. One girl seven months into her first pregnancy arrived in very poor shape with a facial abscess. This was drained, then iron, vitamins and other medication were given as she recovered. When the time came for her drain to be removed, she cried and cried. "Is it painful?" "No. I wonder what would have happened to me if you hadn't come. I am so grateful." Ellen reckoned she would have died.

2007 was a difficult year to plan camps. Elections were due, originally planned for May. Election time is not a good time to be on the road. Then the dates changed and changed again. Eka Dev showed his resilience as Nepali lead. In the end, they were held in November! The June camp was in the most remote place of all, in Mugu district. This was known to be the poorest, least developed of all Nepal's districts. Because food was sufficient for only six months, the government provided some extra food when needed, but the people were at near starvation levels in the cold months. Fears and superstitions were deeply rooted, antenatal care uncommon, delivery was routinely in the goat stable. Typically, mother and baby were not fed for three days, until the mother's milk was 'in'. The infant mortality rate was high and vaccinations rare. Shirley Heywood was the gynaecologist and had been to Mugu in 2001. Little had changed. The local doctor and most of the staff were absent, but the three remaining Nepali nurses were keen to be involved—it was probably a highlight of their time while posted to Mugu. INF had a community development team there, and they gave full help during and after the camp. How important they would become for the breaking down of fear in the longer term, acceptance of vaccines, and health education. There was a darkness about the area.

Dr Sarah Puttix was the anaesthetist both in Rolpa and Mugu. Her father, Graham Scott Brown, had been leader of INF, and, in the 1970s, had trekked extensively in the remote western areas of Nepal, looking for suitable sites for TB and leprosy work. Sarah had grown up in Pokhara. She takes up the story:

"I headed off from Pokhara to Gamgadhi, capital of Mugu. The journey started with a seven-hour drive down to the Terai and along to Nepalganj. Being the hottest time of the year, the air felt like an industrial hair drier blowing through the windows. The temperature was 41.8°C in Nepalganj, where we had to spend two nights, because of the cancellation of the flight bringing the surgeons from Kathmandu. Lying under a fan and mosquito net was an extremely sweaty experience. And there were people working! Even my Minstrel sweets melted into a solid block. With the team complete, we headed up to Surkhet and joined our flight to Mugu.

"The flight was one of the most dramatic experiences of my life. The foothills around Mugu rise to over 12,000 ft, and the plane makes its way through deep valleys and pops over passes with little to spare. It was stunning. We landed on a massive terrace cut into the hillside, with cliffs at either end. [You can get a scary view of Talchaur airstrip on You Tube—Ed]. It was so exciting that my legs trembled for five minutes after leaving the plane!

"We unloaded our gear onto mules and porters, but there was too much stuff, so we had to leave it for the next day. One porter carried the 70 kg generator for the two-and-a-half-hour walk to the hospital. Amazingly, the camp team turned a dirty building into an operating theatre, ultrasound room and outpatient clinic—still dirty but better. Many women walked a long way with prolapses, but then many said no to surgery. This was understandable, as the monsoon was due any day, and field work, especially rice planting, was vital. Post-op rest was not an option. Some did stay for surgery, but they were very frightened. In such malnourished patients, even spinal anaesthetic was difficult, but safer than a general. Being up in Mugu is something else! A person over 40 kg would be thought of as fat, and life expectancy for a woman was 38. There are no toilets. Flies swarm everywhere carrying disease. Most of the team became unwell for a spell.

"On day 2, I really wondered if I was going to be able to hold it all together or if I was going to start crying and never stop. For all the team members who had not been in Mugu before, it was a quite overwhelming experience. Fortunately, clinically all went well. Shirley and Regina, the theatre nurse, stayed overnight in case anyone bled, though we had no idea how to start the generator!

"Shirley saw a number of childless women. Two had no uterus and two no ovaries. Was there inbreeding in this community? Another had never had a period because she was so malnourished. One woman had had 12 children, eight of them stillborn. There were a few, some with gynae problems, others with a mix of problems, who were referred on, with financial help available through the resident INF team. Will any take the opportunity? An 18-month-old child came, seemingly blind. This was clearly Vitamin A deficiency. Not unusual in Nepal. With rehydration and vitamins, it seemed the child was beginning to see—over to the INF nutritionist resident in Mugu.

"One of the ladies came with a long, sad history of a fistula. She had been married at 13, and had her first child, born dead, after a difficult labour which resulted in a fistula. Her husband had left her destitute. She earned a little, carrying heavy loads, and was a social outcaste. Shirley had a policy of referring such patients to Kathmandu or Dharan, but realised this lady could never do that. So, she did a full repair, confident the INF and hospital staff would perform her bladder care.

"Shirley thought, 'There is a fatalism here, probably due to a mixture of religious belief, anaemia (dietary and hookworm), malnutrition and exhaustion in the mothers, and bitter experience'."

The return journey was bittersweet. The team decided to walk to the beautiful Rara Lake, at 9,000 ft. It required a 3,000 ft hot climb, but the compensation was a swim in the lake and a night in a tourist lodge. This is becoming a favourite trekking destination, a two-day walk up from Jumla. The evening was spent around the fire enjoying Nepali folk music. Next day at 5 am, they headed back to the airport, to which all the baggage had been carried the previous day. They waited, then waited again until they heard: "No plane today, the pilot has gone home." There were people at the air ground, which had little accommodation, who had been waiting six days. Eka Dev tried for a helicopter. There was not one that day, but it would come the next. The morning brought the early signs of the monsoon, clouds swathing the hills and rain began to fall. No helicopter. "It seems ridiculous now, but we did begin to wonder if we might be in Mugu for some time. All the hotels were full of people waiting a very long time. Finally, on day three, after five hours of, 'It's coming/it's not coming,' an old Russian helicopter came and whisked us all away through the clouds and back to our normal lives."

What a struggle to help people who weren't sure they wanted help. Only by steady building up of the society, bringing in all types of education, would the people's lives be substantially improved. Compared even to the very poor communities in Doti, Mugu needed much support, being further north and thus more isolated. Later, INF started more projects in some of these mountain regions to offer training to teachers, sponsorship for children from families too poor to pay for education, especially for girls, and provide drinking water, toilets and equipment for schools.

From a camps viewpoint, the policy of reaching out to the very poor seemed right. Maybe greater care was needed in choosing the timing of camps, where the camps team had any say. Going to a remote place in or around the monsoon could result in getting stuck in bad places for weeks, best avoided, as is the extreme heat in the plains. To go to the ends of the earth requires determination!

The first post-monsoon camp was a gynaecology camp in Bajura. The problem was getting there. Roads were damaged by the monsoon. Helicopter trips, from Surkhet, were arranged. Then, late on, a hitch! The senior man in charge of helicopters said they could only take seven people (they hold many more). Was it a safety worry? Discussions went back and forth. In the end, the CDO agreed that this flight was for relief (for the people of Bajura) and rescue (getting the team out)!! The paper was signed. It rained for four days after their arrival, but they got there in good weather. This camp attracted the usual range of women, delighted to have their needs met. Someone had come to look after them!

The great expected event of the year in Nepal was the election. Now the November date had been cancelled. Intense negotiations were ongoing; the Maoists not only held parliamentary seats now but had real power to end the ceasefire. They were holding out for a new constitution and a republic. The struggle with the monarchists continued but the power lay with the Maoists.

It was against the background of this ongoing political instability that camp life went on. Now that there was no November election, with its potential hazards, the desire to go to the poorest could be fulfilled. Two camps were planned, for the first time, one to follow the other, in Kalikot. This is in north-west Nepal. The following description is an excerpt from bossnepal.com:

"It is a district backward in development, education and health. It is very mountainous, 158 miles from Nepalganj, and has one highway, regarded as one of the most treacherous among many in Nepal. Electricity is rare, and people walk everywhere. Nowadays, there is a rough seasonal road and even a bus service. The people living there have a difficult life accessing what most of us take for granted. 75% of the population of 120,000 live between 6,000 and 10,000 ft. The winter snowline in Nepal is at about 8,000 ft."

About 20% of households can only produce food for less than one month per year and struggle to grow rice, maize and wheat on small, steep terraces, with little irrigation. The average monthly income is about £27, which is below the absolute poverty line, as defined by the World Bank.

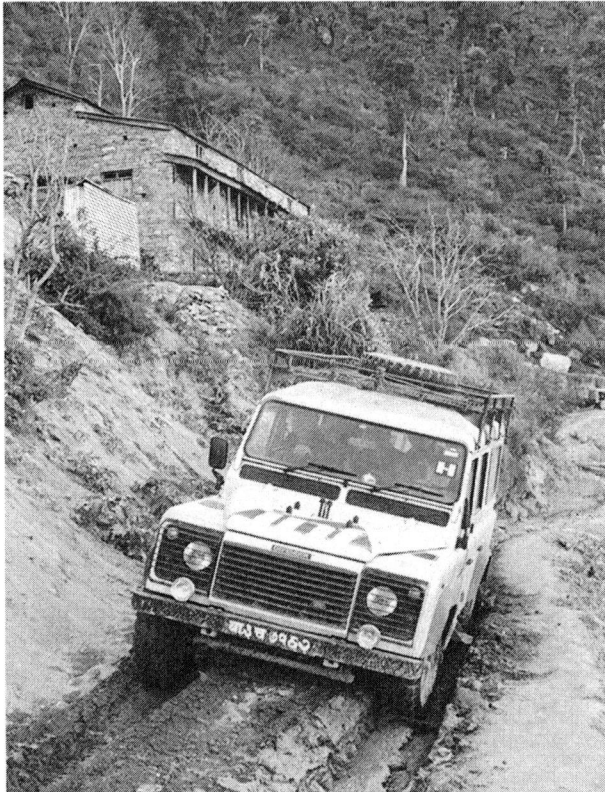

*An INF Land Rover fights its way up to Kalikot.*

The advance party for Kalikot made the road trip and realised this was impossible for the main party. They managed to travel to Surkhet by road, meeting the travelling consultants including Mike Smith and Lukas Eberle.

Unfortunately, this time, the Department for Aviation stuck to the rule of seven persons per flight, meaning two helicopters were needed for the 15-minute flight. There had been a recent helicopter crash, and it seemed the ministry was anxious in case a flight full of foreigners met a similar fate! However, as it turned out, the helicopter was packed tight with locals alongside the seven team members!

This Kalikot ear camp, for the first time, met opposition from an unexpected quarter. Medicins Sans Frontières (MSF) were working in Kalikot, and they questioned the camp team's capability to fulfil its mission. Some seemed threatened by another team arriving on their turf. They resisted the use of 'their' beds and paramedical staff. Meetings were held, but they were reluctant to do as requested by the District Medical Officer. Camps are always pre-arranged with the local health and government authorities and local staff, who were very co-operative in Kalikot. During the camp, the team were able to help the young MSF doctors amputate a patient's crushed toe, and trust was restored. There was a sign above the ward door indicating that guns were not to be brought inside; the civil war was very active here too.

Camp got under way. At the end, in her report, Ellen wrote a gross understatement: "There was no shortage of patients, and we were not able to operate on all who needed surgery." All who came to outpatients were seen—1,184 patients—massive numbers of needy people. Many had vitamin deficiencies, particularly B vitamins, resulting in the 'jum jums' — neurological discomfort and tingling in hands and feet. The audiology team was kept busy. The surgeons worked incredibly hard, performing 127 operations, most taking over two hours. All this was achieved in eight working days. And there was still unfinished work. Patients queued, sleeping outside overnight in the cold. That camp looked at one small spectrum, one health need. How much more was needed?

Surgeon Alan Johnson and anaesthetist Charlie Collins shared a room with Mike Smith in the primitive guest house. Each night Alan and Mike were woken as Charlie used his flip-flop to try to scare away the rats that were running on the plastic sheeting nailed to the ceiling above his bed.

One evening, as the surgeons and nurses did their ward round, they met a poor man, caring for his small son after his ear surgery. The boy lay on his mat on the floor. The team asked if he had food. Dad produced a few dried burnt chapatis from his bag and said yes, no problem. He had clearly brought them all the way from his village to sustain them. Such strong and honourable people.

Alan wrote "I very much enjoyed the experience of the camp. The common purpose, fantastic organisation by the Nepali team and 'Super Didi' (Ellen), Mike's energy, Charlie's humour, Philippa Seal's (anaesthetist) smile, Lukas' Swiss chocolates, to name a few, plus the hard work and enthusiasm of all involved and the tolerance of our patients, were all inspirational. Working in such a beautiful place, for remarkable people, was a great opportunity and challenge." Other volunteers included some who came repeatedly, for nursing (such as Carmel Glennie with her lovely Irish accent, bringing boxes of discarded but useful medical items), audiologists like Mike Sanders and his wife Bex from New Zealand, and sometimes a general practitioner. On the return journey, crowds had gathered on the road. The previous day, a child had been killed by a truck and as often happened, the driver continued without stopping, scared for his own life. The poor locals, who built shacks, small shops and houses right on the road, and let their children roam, stopped all the vehicles and demanded compensation for the family. Very sad situations with multiple causes and no easy answers. They had put burning tyres and wood across the road. The team had to get down, carry their bags around the roadblock and eventually managed to hire a minibus on the other side, and continue.

There were a few days break before the surgical camp began, led again by Ian Bissett, (as always, with his wife, Jo who came to make sure he didn't overwork!), and his team from New Zealand, where, in 2016, Ian would be appointed Professor of Surgery in Auckland. The Nepali staff were well cared for in the hospital accommodation, whilst the expatriates stayed in The White House, white on the outside only! It was a difficult walk from the hospital and bitterly cold, with rats running everywhere. "Washing was a luxury!"

For Dr Ian Ferrer, a GP who had previously worked with INF in Pokhara, this was his first of several camps. He remembers feeling colder there than he had ever been before. One of the obvious problems which arose from having a narrow focus, such as surgical, ear and gynaecology camps, is that all sorts of people with other medical problems turn up, hoping for help. Camps often had a general practitioner present. Where simple examination and medication was adequate, these patients were treated by the GP. Others were screened and referred on to the specialists at the camp. Some were seen with major but not urgent surgical problems, like burns contractures, hare lips, or major prostate symptoms. These cases were referred, usually to Pokhara, which by now had several well-equipped hospitals. The local doctors were very relieved to have such problems taken out of their hands.

Again, helicopters had to bring and return staff. That expense was a discouragement to returning there. They were swamped by patients, most of whom would have been better treated in health posts. Patients needing surgery were slow to come at first. The new District Health Officer arrived, and he and his staff triaged 534 patients, referring as necessary to the INF team, who also saw another 882 people. A whole range of problems were seen, the most common being sore bellies, resulting from Giardia and worms; there was also vitamin deficiency, and hookworm anaemia—all of which are endemic in rural Nepal. The MSF lab was helpful for diagnosis. There was some major surgery. Facilities were seriously limited, especially for anaesthetics and blood transfusions and a range of lab tests, in this very cold, very poor, remote place. If a surgeon got into difficulties, there was no intensive care, no major hospital to refer to. This was it! Ultrasound was vitally useful. The surgeons performed a nephrectomy, thyroidectomy, gall bladder removal, mastectomy and Caesarian sections, which probably saved the lives of two mothers and their babies. One man had borrowed £160, eight months wages, to take his wife to Nepalganj. No joy there, so he brought her to this camp, where the surgeons removed a 5 kg ovarian cyst. There were hernia repairs and many haemorrhoids, which were usually treated by being 'banded', with a tight rubber band to shrink them. Several had bladder stones removed; these are common where people drink too little and are repeatedly dehydrated.

Colin Wilson, a surgeon from New Zealand, who attended many camps with Ian, wrote: "I will never forget one early morning walk, when a goatherd, bursting with smiles, left his goats and came up to greet Ian respectfully with 'Namaskar'. 48 hours previously, he had had a repair of a large rectal prolapse and he was so happy to be able to work again."

Colin also recalls a five-year-old boy, who had a stone stuck in his ureter, causing hydronephrosis, a serious kidney problem. "He had suffered repeated attacks of left-sided kidney infection. The diagnosis had been established in India, and his father had his records carefully protected in a clear folder. This father had sold his inherited land and, with the 30,000 rupees from this sale, was carrying his son to the hospital in Nepalganj, about 200km away. As he just happened to be passing by this health post on his journey, he stopped off to ask if the doctors here could help.

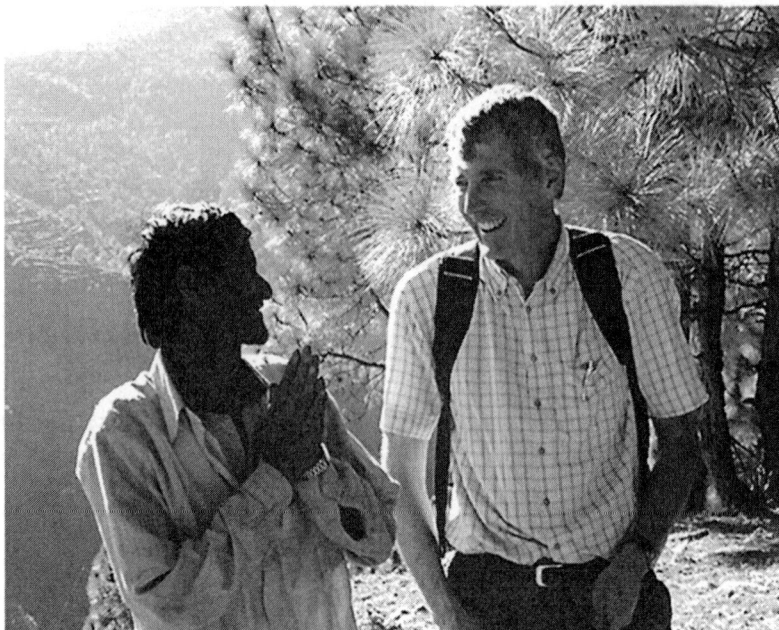

*Ian meets a grateful goatherd on the way to the hospital.*

"The child was quite unwell from the obstructed and infected kidney. The doctors were uncertain whether or not to tackle this procedure in such a remote setting but, after the ultrasound scan was repeated and the diagnosis confirmed, they decided they were prepared to do it. It required a general anaesthetic, opening the bladder and slitting the lower part of the ureter to extract the stone. It proved to be a challenging procedure, but with careful dissection, a pea-sized calculus was teased out of the obstructed ureter, followed by a flood of infected urine. They left a tiny catheter in the ureter for the resident doctor to remove after two weeks. Now there was hope for full recovery. One memorable feature of this operation was not only the skill of the surgeon, but also his extreme patience with the faulty old diathermy machine, which was used to stop the bleeding!"

Colin also recalled "An elderly woman was carried in a doko (a traditional basket carried on the back) for three days to get to the surgical camp. She looked skeletal and deeply jaundiced. An ultrasound scan of her liver showed an obstructed bile duct and an inoperable cancer. The surgeons advised against her going down to India to look for treatment, as this would deplete her loving family of their meagre finances, with little or no benefit. Ellen was able to explain this sensitively to them and the advice was readily accepted. They returned to their remote village, knowing the reality of this sad news, but encouraged by Ellen's words of comfort."

MSF had allocated 10 beds. They were all full by the second day; post-op patients then recovered on the floor. Nepal Red Cross and the army came up with mats and blankets, not all of which were returned! At times, it was mind-blowing to see the depth of need.

Ian Ferrer recalls the return journey, from Kalikot to Surkhet: "The old Russian helicopter was overloaded with equipment and the camps team. The airstrip was carved into the cliff. The helicopter struggled to leave the ground and the pilot flew to the edge of the airstrip, only three feet off the ground. The helicopter then suddenly dropped 1,000 feet down towards the valley, at which altitude, the rotors found sufficient air to bring it under control. We returned safely to Surkhet, but I had been thinking we were definitely going to die!"

MSF had arranged a much-needed gynaecology camp for six months later on. This seems like the tip of the iceberg. What is the answer? Certainly, occasional camps will meet some people's big need, and that is good. Local health posts play a crucial role if properly staffed and equipped. They will become increasingly effective, providing ante-natal and maternity services, vaccinations and under-five care, along with health education, not least in schools. These will probably save more lives than anything else. In Nepal, the government is progressively rolling out these services. INF also contributes to the improvements with training projects for Nepali women volunteers in remote communities to deliver vital maternal and child healthcare. They learn how to care for mothers and babies during the 'Golden 1,000 Days' between conception and the child's second birthday. Fortified food for babies helps to improve the under-five mortality and severe malnutrition, which would result in poor health and disability.

District hospitals need more trained staff to enable them to diagnose and treat some of the patients who come to surgical and gynaecology camps. Massive infrastructure is harder to come by: safe roads and airports, water, electricity, sanitation, adequate food. It is a big task for a government faced with widespread poverty, impossible if there is unrest.

# Chapter 17

## 2008: A Tumultuous Year

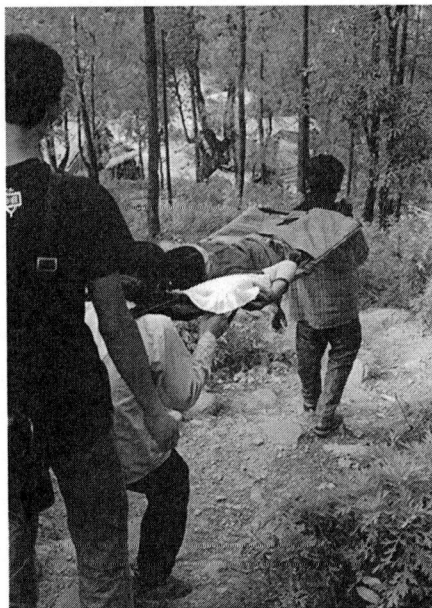

*A patient being carried home from hospital.*

Ellen returned to Nepal on January 31, to make full use of her five-month visa. Three early camps had been arranged, the first in the very isolated district of Dailekh, starting within two days of her landing. She needed to adjust again to what promised to be a rigorous time. The Nepali team had done all the preparation and were ready to go. Ellen's role was to ensure the consultant specialists were organised and briefed. There was more to that than is immediately obvious. They might never have been to a developing country before. What to bring? Toilet paper, bedding, food treats, warm or cold weather clothes? This became such a repetitive task for Mike Smith, who always brought a group with him, that he and a friend, Mike Falter, eventually put it all onto a website for people to consult. Having said and done all that, nothing can quite prepare a person for the shock of rural Nepal. Amazingly perhaps, only one doctor was unable to cope and that was in the extreme conditions in Mugu. Faced with enormous challenges, the warmth and friendliness of the team won through.

Dailekh District is in the middle range of hills in Mid-West Nepal, with a population of about 250,000. In 2008, there was no tarmac road and no airport; in other words, you walked. It is said that, as in Mugu, 80% of the population were subsistence farmers, and for many, the food lasted for only six months of the year. One of the extraordinary facts about Nepal is that so many people have lived for centuries in remote places. What a task for a government to develop these areas. Inevitably, the forests are cut down for fuel. Deforestation leads to lethal landslides and destruction of arable land. All these privations make it particularly difficult for the women in the community to get any treatment. The gynaecology camp held in Dailekh was therefore of enormous benefit.

A plastic surgery camp was held in early April in another remote district of the medieval kingdom of Doti. Many there retain their own language—Dotyali. Local interpreters have to be found. A smaller team was assembled for this camp.

Political events continued to develop. 2008 was a year of tumultuous change for Nepal. Elections were eventually held after several false starts. This was a nation in political turmoil. In the 18th century Prithvi Narayan Shah from Gorkha subdued many small kingdoms to unify Nepal. Then the Rana family established a system of hereditary prime ministers until a monarchy was reinstated in 1951, when King Tribhuvan, a descendant of Prithvi Narayan Shah came to power. In 1959 his son king Mahendra took over and established a pyramidal Panchayat system of government with himself as the head of state. During most of these periods Nepal had a policy of isolation from the outside world, which was intended as a defence against colonial powers but also led to lack of development. After an attempt at establishing parliamentary democracy in 1959 and another in 1990, came civil war and several unstable governments, with further confusion caused by the murder of most members of the royal family in 2001. Nepal had been the world's only Hindu Kingdom, (although it also had a large Buddhist population, and significant numbers of Muslims in some districts).

The people were unable to make their wishes known, and the country continued to develop very slowly. This lack of development and support for the poor was what the Maoist uprising was all about. King Gyanendra tried to wrest back power in 2005 but the Maoists were having none of it. Fighting escalated before peace talks took place. It was decided that Nepal would become a secular state with a parliamentary democracy, described as Nepal's Magna Carta, a charter for human rights.

Following this, with the Maoists in the discussion, came the debate on how Parliament was to be established. Eventually, a first-past-the-post system was agreed for 220 seats, proportional representation for 330 seats and appointees to 26 seats. At that point, finally, elections were held, generally peacefully. To everyone's surprise, the Maoists won 38% of the 601 seats. Prachanda, the Maoist leader, became Prime Minister, and it was decided he would go to the king and tell him he was no longer king and must leave his palace, though he could return to life as an ordinary citizen, which he did!

Thus ended 240 years of monarchy. It also ended the status of Nepal as a Hindu state. To be part of the United Nations, that change, to freedom of religion, was necessary. There was a backlash. A Hindu movement arose in Eastern Nepal, more bombs were let off and some of the funds were raised by terrorising the many small Nepali churches, demanding money.

Against this background, INF camps continued. It needed more than a Maoist revolution or a profound political change to shake Ellen Findlay from her avowed intent to bring health, compassion and care to the downtrodden, forgotten people of Nepal. Health professionals continued to come from across the globe to bring help in beautiful but desperate places, often cold, sometimes hot, always uncomfortable, with dubious food. How well the Nepali team had done in those dangerous years, and how grateful they were that no one came to harm.

The biannual ear camp was moved from Achham back to Dailekh. Site change was easy enough, given time but dates were fixed, as visiting consultants and GPs had booked leave and flights. Volunteers all paid their own way, and most took annual leave, a sacrifice for their families. Sometimes, their home hospital would grant some of the leave as study time; it was certainly a learning curve! Encountering and treating advanced stages of disease and working alongside Nepali colleagues in a completely different health delivery environment presented multiple challenges. As before, access to Dailekh was very difficult—what must it be like for local people with no financial resources! Helicopters were again necessary to bring the team and equipment. But the rewards were great. Trust had been built, and people came from everywhere. Mike and his team were inundated, with 150 operations. As usual, there were non-ear-related problems, such as a woman who had had a large lump in her neck for years, which turned out to be tuberculosis following biopsy, and thus treatable. The audiology teams were getting bigger and busier, with 450 hearing tests and teaching 100 patients how to use their hearing aids, care for them and obtain spares. Alice, the dentist, attended again and treated 130 people.

A man brought his wife to the gynaecology camp and also their only son. The child had a cleft palate. Ellen told them that there would be a plastic surgery camp shortly, saw they were very poor, and offered to pay the debts caused by coming to this camp. As she counted out different denominations of Nepali rupees, his eyes boggled. He had never seen so many different notes. Ellen also offered to put him in a 'hotel' until his wife was fit to travel, "Oh, I couldn't do that. I am a high caste Brahmin. I cannot stay in another caste's hotel or eat their food."

The caste system, a 3,000-year-old social structure in Hinduism, is rigid. The high caste (Brahmins) are the academic experts in Hindu law and the intellectuals. Next in rank are the warrior castes, then the workers, and finally the untouchables, those who work with animal skin to make leather, and sweep and clean up, including latrines. It is your lot (karma) in life and is fixed. Two big changes have seriously challenged these Hindu customs. First, the availability of education: as young people mix in schools and colleges, so the barriers begin to break down. However, the structure remains strong in the rural areas and also when it comes to marriage and funerals. The second challenge which Nepal is having to face is the result of the political upheaval of 2008. In the former Hindu state, the king was a manifestation of a Hindu god, 'five times holy, king of kings', but now he is an ordinary citizen. Nepal is declared a secular state, with many freedoms, including that of religion. No wonder there has been a backlash from militant Hindus! Despite the declaration of a secular state, the legal code still includes provisions for criminal prosecution and even imprisonment if someone is accused of trying to change another person's religion from that of their parents.

Perhaps surprisingly, with the risk of violent storms at the end of the monsoon, the camp returned to Lamjung. One of the earliest camps had been held there in the monsoon, with enormous travel difficulties. Mid-September is just about alright. It is a time of intense activity in the fields, preparing for the rice harvest in October. Despite the essential fieldwork taking precedence, this gynaecology camp was as busy as usual, in a very pleasant climate. One of the specialists had experience in repairing vesicovaginal fistulas. Knowing this skill was available, the camp was advertised on Nepal Radio with information about this huge problem and about the camp. People even came from the east of the country to the small, isolated Lamjung hospital.

Inevitably, with this continuous workload, equipment wore out and needed replacement. Two gifts were received and new equipment ordered. The vehicles took a pounding on the Nepali roads. An extraordinary gift of £30,000 was given for vehicles by one of the visiting surgeons, enabling the team to buy two replacement vehicles. Money was never solicited. Information was disseminated through Ellen's newsletters, and networking of volunteers. Many would return home and raise money through Rotary clubs, churches or sponsored activities. Some would collect and donate items of medical equipment, dressings, or hearing aids.

Ellen said: "It was hard work getting to the Awalching ear camp. The 'road' left much to be desired. Even the tough Nepali buses didn't tackle the road up to Awalching. The Regional Medical Officer had supplied two jeeps to help with transport on this four-hour journey. It was a pleasure to disgorge from the vehicles, organise porters and walk down the hillside for an hour to the health centre. As I walked along, I wondered where the patients would come from. There were hardly any houses to be seen as our walk twisted down the hill between the scattered small farm buildings and animals. I needn't have worried. On the first morning, 320 patients were waiting to register!

"This camp in Awalching was a last-minute change. It had been arranged for Surkhet, but the hospital there made it clear that a charge would be made for each operation, from the camp funds to the hospital. Hmmm!

"It was the Regional Director of Health, Dr Ananda Shrestha, again, who offered Awalching as an alternative to Surkhet. He was clearly glad, as were the local officials and MPs, who planned an opening ceremony. Everything to make our stay as comfortable as possible was arranged and paid for by the Regional Director's office, including adequate accommodation and food, porterage and the two jeeps. The local committee ensured sufficient water was available as well as furniture. Patients were provided with blankets and sleeping mats. There was no electricity, so our generator was used during operations. Whilst such hospitality had been known before, it was rare. Was this a fruit of the new politics? Time would tell. The sleeping accommodation was in an unused part of the health centre, on metal hospital beds with no mattresses. Three of the surgeons and one anaesthetist 'slept' in one small room, and each time one turned over in his sleep, the sheet metal of the bed rattled and woke the others. There was no hotel, so all food was prepared outdoors and cooked in a huge cauldron, on an open fire."

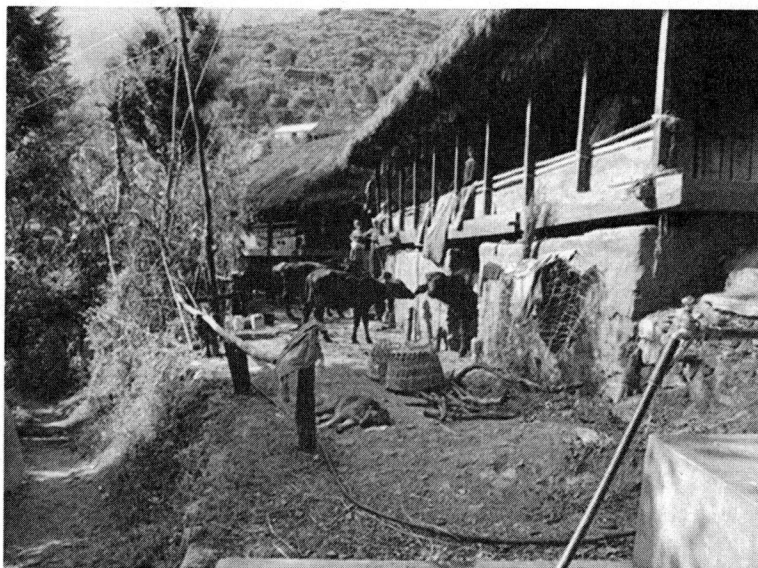

*A typical farmhouse in the scattered hillside community of Awalching.*

Despite the seeming remoteness, patients appeared from a wide area. Camp must have seemed a remarkable event to local people. Five consultants from UK and other staff all gathered in this remote village spread across the side of a steep valley, to operate on them and bring hearing aids. The team saw, assessed and treated well over 1,000 patients. Unusually, three patients had large parotid salivary gland tumours removed, from just in front of the ear. It was quite a day, three patients having their parotid surgery, side by side on the simple operating tables. This operation can leave the face muscles on that side paralysed, so great care is needed, to preserve the facial nerve. The other interesting feature in outpatients was several people with enlarged thyroid glands (goitres) indicating a lack of iodine in the area. Oddly, unless the goitre was very large and getting in the way, many women (who are much more affected than men) liked to keep them, as they are seen as good luck!

As always, there were patients with treatable conditions, but they had to be referred to other centres because there was no post-op care or facilities available. One man had had his ear operated on by Mike on a previous camp far away in western Nepal. He heard the radio announcement that always preceded the camps and travelled to this village in order to have his other ear fixed.

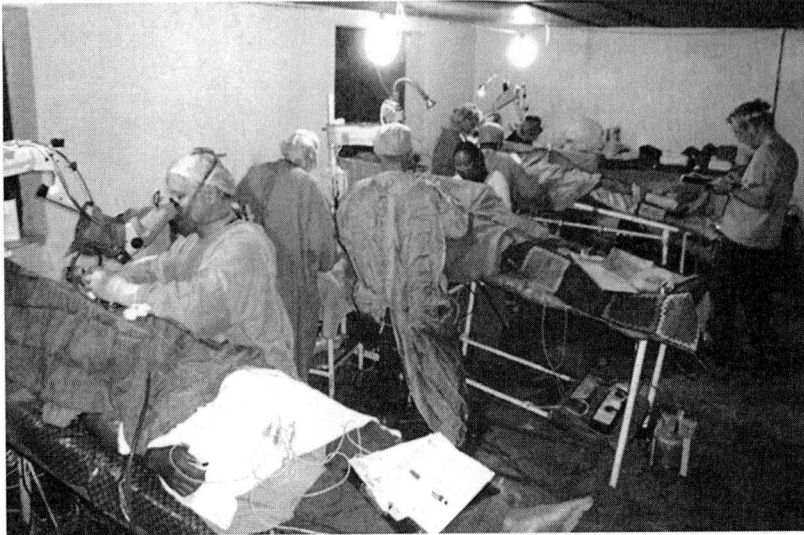

*The operating room set up in Awalching.*

Ellen said: "Mike is amazing and will go to any lengths to help a patient. A man came with a huge nasal polyp, filling the nose and back of the throat. He had had it removed several times before but here he was again, hardly able to breathe. Mike agreed to operate. I went into the theatre when the man was on the table. Charlie, the anaesthetist, whispered to me 'Mike cannot find the bleeding point. It is torrential, from far back in the nasal cavity' I went out and prayed, returning five minutes later. All was under control. Mike said 'I couldn't find the bleeder and then suddenly the bleeding stopped, and I could see what to do.'"

One of our anaesthetists, Paddy, had studied navigation by the stars, for his sailing qualification. The village had almost no light pollution, so we sat in the evenings and looked at the brilliant sky, all the clearer because of our altitude. No machinery, no roads; silence, and a clear sky. Paddy pointed out the faint smudges of the nebula in Orion's sword, and the galaxy of Andromeda. Many shooting stars could be seen at this time of year. On another camp someone brought binoculars, and they could see planets and even the moons of Jupiter.

The hour's walk back up the hill to the road reminded Ellen that her hips were wearing out. She needed anti-inflammatory tablets to keep her going, but camp had gone well.

146

Some of the team went on to trek in the Langtang valley north of Kathmandu, an area that was sadly devastated a few years later by a major earthquake and landslide, which wiped out the small village of Langtang that lay below the magnificent Langtang mountain and its glacier.

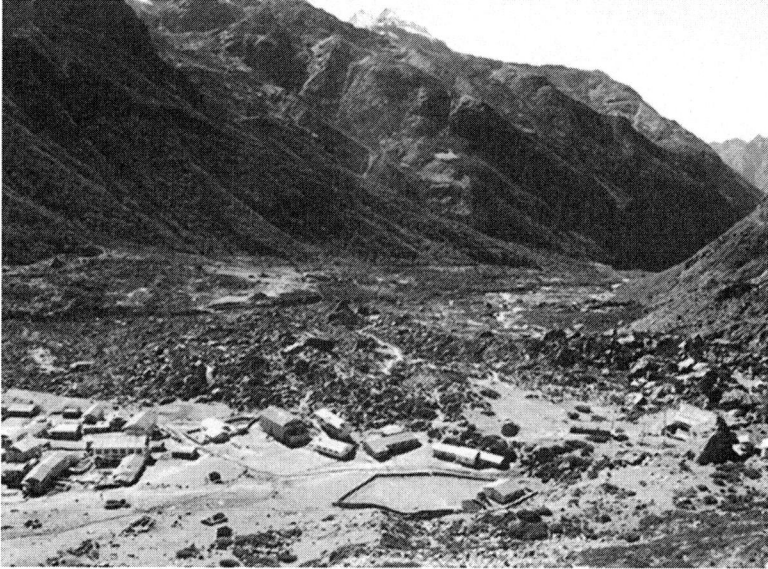

*Langtang village.*

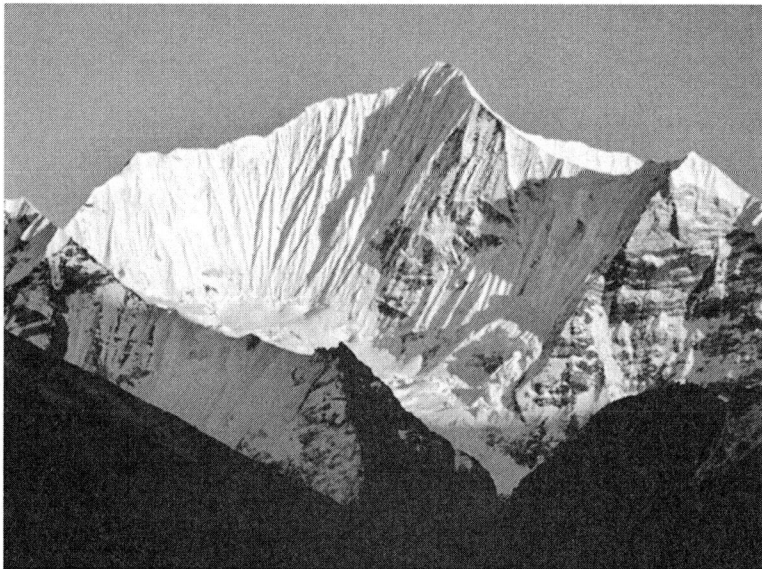

*Langtang Himal, rising above the Langtang valley.*

# Chapter 18

## To Bajhang and Bajura

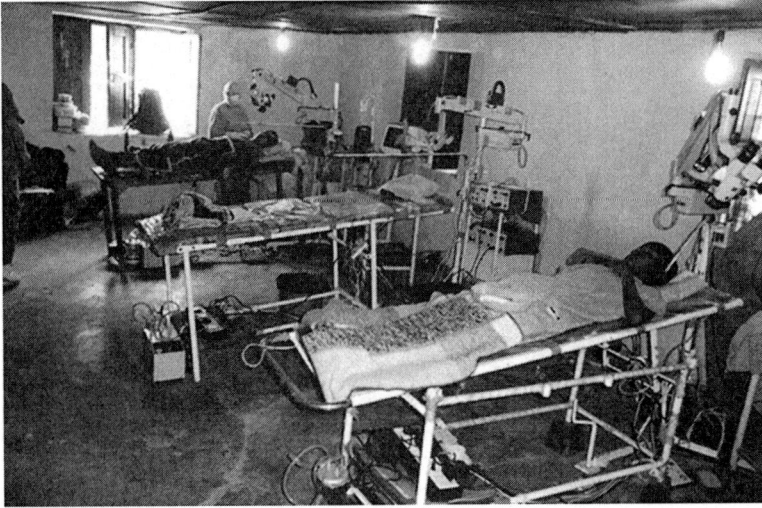

*Typical operating room set up for an ear camp.*

During the first camp of 2009, the team was visited by the Regional Director of Health, who looked at the health promotion leaflets, in the Nepali language, which they had been giving out to patients. "The government are now beginning to think about such leaflets," he said. "Can I take some of these to the Health Minister in Kathmandu?"

The government had decided they would like to acknowledge the work of camps. Two days before the event was due to take place, the Regional Director was called away. "Just as well," Ellen wrote. "As we were preparing to come down from the hills, the heavens opened and rain lashed down, preventing us from travelling. It took us six hours to get there and 12 hours coming back on the mud-sliding roads." It had been a good camp, excellent team, many patients and warm weather, until the downpour at the end.

Ellen wrote home to her supporters about individual patients:

"The 11-year-old girl with incontinence whom we referred has had her surgery in Kathmandu and is cured. She said, 'When I get married, I will send you an invitation.' Marriage later on would now be possible. A couple who had no children after seven years was now expecting, after treatment.

"There were sad stories too. A young girl had been married a year but no child yet. So her husband left her. Another man said he would take her, and if they had children he would marry her. If not, he would look for someone else. She was so unhappy. Another woman came with a lump the size of a football on her knee. We referred her to a good orthopaedic surgeon in Pokhara and paid her bills. It turned out to be cancerous, with secondaries in the lung. We continued to give her support."

Bajhang District borders Tibet, where a trade route runs through the high Himalayas. Nearly 200,000 people live in Bajhang, extraordinary for such a high remote area with no road. The large number of people who live in isolated, poverty-stricken areas makes Nepal a very special target for development funds. It is said that 30% live above 15,000 ft, hard to believe.

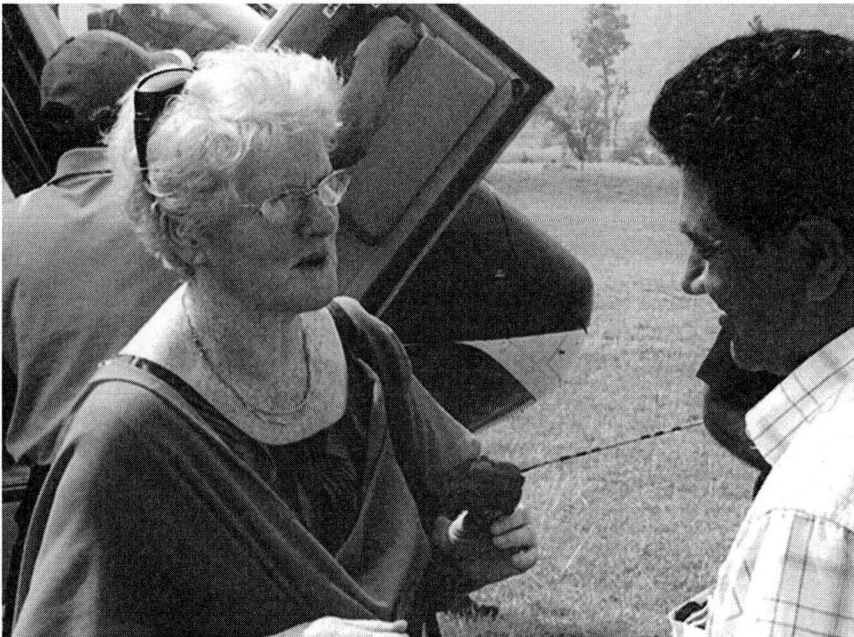

*Sister Ellen discusses travel plans.*

Ellen tells the story of the camp:

"Getting there for the ear camp was challenging. We had to hope the big helicopter was working. It wasn't! We shuttled up from Nepalganj (to which the visiting team had flown) in five trips in the little helicopter. Even then, I

149

wondered if we would get out again. Living was in accommodation with one toilet between the 17 of us, and a shower room with no electricity! But the scenery in Bajhang was stunningly beautiful and made up for all the inconveniences.

"Bajhang is poor and the people appreciated the care given. While I was walking home with a patient's relative one night, he said, 'We've never seen a camp like this before. Can you come and do a women's camp?'

"The hospital was filthy, toilets unusable. I never saw the floors being washed. Indeed, the person responsible was more involved in nursing care. Nurses were in short supply." The bedbugs were the worst they had encountered! Mike put a nylon poncho over his cotton mattress, sprayed it each night with repellant, and crept into his sheet sleeping bag, tied at the top, with just his nose pointing out to breathe!

Why were there so many ear camps? In part, this was down to availability. Mike Smith was an ENT consultant, and the contract he negotiated in UK allowed him to come twice yearly. He had contact with other specialists, such as ENT surgeons, anaesthetists, audiologists and theatre nurses. The other reason is that ear disease is extremely common in Nepal. Many patients have chronic smelly, discharging and often deaf ears. This is probably due to a combination of factors such as lack of cleanliness, genetic predisposition, malnutrition, vitamin deficiencies, wood smoke in homes with poor ventilation, frequent runny noses and colds in children and lack of appropriate use (and availability) of antibiotics. One young girl at this camp had pus coming not just from the ear but also from the mastoid bone behind the ear. She would soon have developed meningitis. Surgery went well, and she was restored to health and hearing. Such patients were not uncommon. Profound deafness from birth or early childhood is also much commoner than in more developed countries. Most of those affected grow up to be deaf and dumb, using limited sign language.

For the first time, three anaesthetists were available for the three surgeons, and there were three operating tables! Sometimes patients, whilst not feeling pain, were aware of the noise of the drill delicately clearing away infected bone from the mastoid, which was disturbing for them. Because it was both sedating and a powerful painkiller, Ketamine could be king! After he had finished, the anaesthetist, having supervised sedation and safety throughout, was responsible for ensuring immediate post-op care—no recovery rooms, oxygen or monitoring here, though such equipment was increasingly available to the camps team, mainly through donations of used items. As the team expanded, the weight of equipment needed rose from 300 kgs in the early days, past 600 kgs, up to 1,200 kgs, all of which had to be transported.

A girl came with what at first was thought to be a foreign body in her eye. In fact, the front of her eye had been perforated by something sharp, and when the team discovered that there was an eye hospital not far over the border, in India, the patient was sent there.

The last day of any busy camp was hard. After changing dressings, discharging patients, clearing the hospital and packing up, the exhausted teams hoped desperately that the helicopter would arrive!

Up at 7 am to walk to the airstrip for the 9 am flight. It had to fly over three districts. Cloud cover in one area prevented flying. 3 pm came and went. If it didn't come…. but in the end, it did (the next day) which meant another night in the 'hotel' with the bed bugs! That was especially hard for the weary visitors who were looking forward to a comfortable bed that night! The team arrived in Nepalganj, to find a strike, with only rickshaws available, taking a chance to charge higher than their normal rates. It was quite a sight! Limited rickshaws, big suitcases and heavy foreigners aboard, trying to get to half-decent hotels—no wonder the rickshaw wallahs charged more! "It was wonderful to get back to civilisation, a lovely shower and decent food." That, at any rate, was Ellen's view. I don't think many visitors would rate Nepalganj quite like that—a hot, dusty, noisy border town. But after Bajhang, maybe it seemed very good.

The fun wasn't yet finished. Roads were blocked, taxis on strike. Locals had laid burning tyres and wood across the road. Eventually after some phone calls, they were able to call a minibus to meet them on the other side, having carried their bags around the roadblock. The Maoists were flexing their muscles again. The reason? The government army was not prepared to take the Maoist army members into its ranks, hardly surprising as they had been killing each other for ten years. One problem was that these rebel soldiers needed work, or they might just find another cause to fight for. Eventually that inclusion would happen, but for now chaos reigned. However, planes usually continued to fly during strikes, so the visitors were able to get back to Kathmandu. The Nepali team flew two days later, but trying to get to Pokhara by road, they were blocked again and had to take a circuitous route, and return via Kathmandu. How easy to blockade this country with so few roads!

The truck carrying all the equipment had an accident when the roads were clear again. No injuries but a £900 bill for repairs. The Nepali team said, "This has been the most difficult camp of all to organise." What a terrific, often unnoticed, job they did, absolutely vital now that Ellen was spending less time in Nepal.

Because of the difficulty of the Bajhang camp, it was decided to hold the three post-monsoon camps all in Bajura: first an ear camp, then gynaecology, finishing with a surgical camp. This had never been tried before. It would mean the main team being away for six weeks, bringing in three separate teams of specialists. Rural Nepal had never had such a range of specialists, all within a few weeks. This was not going to be easy! Bajura is geographically split into three zones: very high mountains, high mountains, and mid mountains, with a deprived population of 135,000, many living above 6,000 ft. There were plans for a road but nothing ready yet. There were several secondary schools. Nevertheless, the literacy rate in all these remote mountainous regions was estimated at 32%, meaning health leaflets with lots of pictures and repeated verbal explanations were essential.

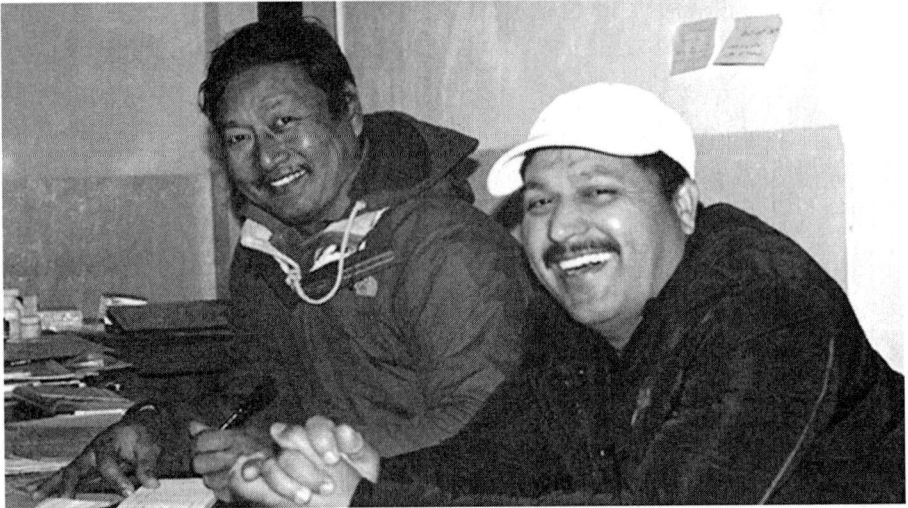

*Rabi Gurung, biotechnician; and Eka Dev, co-ordinator.*

As Ellen prepared for these three camps, she wrote of her appreciation of her Nepali team:

Eka Dev Devkota, the camps co-ordinator.

Robin Lama, operating theatre-in-charge.

Rabi Gurung our technician who ensures all the equipment works well.

Anandi, Ganga, and Indra ensure cleanliness and availability of equipment for the doctors and surgeons, absolutely crucial!

Regina Thapa* and Dil Kumari, scrub nurses who join us for camps.

The four drivers, with a hard task, who also fetch and carry and organise patients at camp.

Regina's story is a wonderful one:

> "Dr Ruth Watson's chief help in theatre in the Shining Hospital, Pokhara, was Regina. She had come, orphaned, from a village many miles away. Dr and Mrs Turner employed her initially as their cook. She had had no education but learnt well. After a while, she went up to the Shining Hospital to do her nursing training. Many village girls with little formal education were accepted for training, giving them hope for useful employment, and Regina was one such. She did so well that, after her two years' training, Ruth took her into theatre and trained her in sterilising, recognising instruments, laying up tables for surgery, cleaning away afterwards and being the main assistant at most cases. Her help was invaluable. When it seemed the government might close the Shining Hospital, Regina, with others, began morning school (from 6:00–9:00 am) to increase her education, and when she had attained a sufficient standard, she went off to begin government training. The years of expertise she had gained counted for nothing. As with other girls, the Shining's loss was the government's gain." [1]

Here she was, 40 years later, still serving her people.

Ellen wrote: "There were only three days between finishing the Bajura ear and gynae camps and starting the surgical one, with a new set of visiting consultants. Fortunately, we returned to Surkhet to rest for a few days, but then when we wanted to return to Bajura we were told that the big helicopter was out of action again and we would need to do five flights in the smaller one. There was no other option, as there was no road access. How would the funds stand up to this? But it was worth every penny for the number of lives that benefitted. We were overloaded again.

---

[1] Hawker, David *Kanchi Doctor (Updated): Ruth Watson of Nepal*, Available from Amazon Kindle.

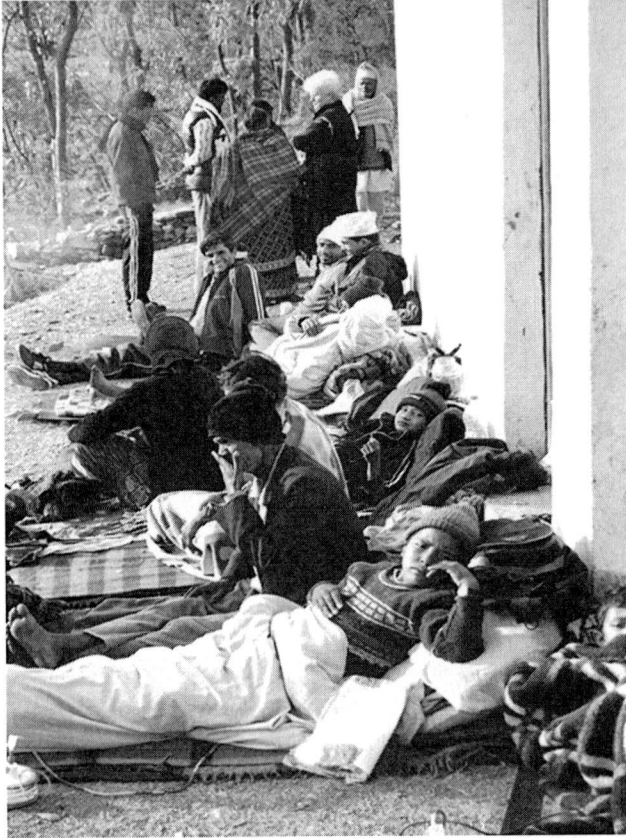

*Surgical patients recover in the sun outside the small district hospital in Bajura.*

"One woman had had an abdominal lump for 19 years. When removed, the cyst weighed 7.5kg, our biggest yet! Patients from previous camps came to show us how well they were. But there were many unmet needs and the hope was to return again." Ellen concluded, "These camps were in remote areas with poor access. There was no electricity, so again we had to use our generator during surgery. Some patients had walked five days and had suffered their problems for many years. It was a privilege for us to serve them, bringing physical relief, love and compassion".

The three camps went smoothly. More patients with cancer were seen here than was usual, including lung cancer. Most Nepalis smoked, homes were often polluted with wood smoke, and in Kathmandu, traffic pollution is amongst the worst in the world. Smoking began in the 1960s in a big way. Typically, lung cancer occurs after 40 years of smoking. It was about to become a big problem in Nepal. Thankfully tobacco advertising has now been banned.

During the 30 days of work, there were 3,099 outpatients and 384 operations were performed, plus many ultrasounds, hearing tests and hearing aid fittings. Sixteen patients were referred on, and fifteen of these made their way to Nepalganj, Pokhara or Kathmandu, all four-day journeys. All fifteen had vital surgery. One had chemo and radiotherapy with good results. "One of the cancer patients didn't believe we would pay all his expenses and sold land and animals to raise the money. We will try to buy them back as he is a widower with children—the land was their inheritance."

Many of the hill people are animists, appeasing and fearing evil spirits. This is mingled with Hinduism. Ellen experienced an alarming event, one she had seen several times before, well-recognised by the locals. "One morning there was a lot of shouting. It sounded like a man, but it was a woman possessed by an evil spirit. She was spitting, snarling and shouting, and was not being helped by her male relatives, who were provoking her, thinking they could drive out the spirit. When I got to the woman, a local medicine man was stuffing rice grains and tobacco into her mouth to get rid of the spirit. The family explained that there was an evil spirit roaming round their village. The local witchdoctor was able to get rid of the spirit, but it moved to another person. This woman had gone at 4 am to milk the buffalo when the spirit came onto her. We offered to pray for her and explained that the spirit would leave her. The family were dubious but we took the woman inside and quietly prayed. The woman became quiet, then fell asleep. The surprised family took her home."

This situation is not uncommon in village Nepal. Wikipedia, commenting on Bajura, says, "For emergency medical care people need to travel to the district centre or Kathmandu. Many just die. People still believe in the *Dhami* or *Jankri* (witchdoctors)."

It is clear that Ellen's strength and resilience came from her Christian faith. She would often pray with anxious or terminally ill people. At camp, she would gather those who wished in the morning for a short 'thought for the day and prayer'.

Ellen accepted all who were willing to come to work on camp, based only on expertise. One visiting surgeon wrote to her on his return: "Not only was Nepal one of the very best highlights of my year, it was one of the most rewarding experiences of my life, not least for meeting all of you, but also because I have never spent any time with anyone who had such faith. Ellen and Peggy (Franks), you have made a very hardcore, atheist surgeon much more

155

reflective. Indeed, many of my close acquaintances, whilst recognising it is a change for the better, have been a little concerned about how radical it has been after just a fortnight away with you all. At times when things get out of hand at work, I think of you guys and my teeny experience of what you do in Nepal, and it makes me feel better. If you will have me again, I would dearly love to come back."

Another wrote: "I am still trying to get the two weeks in Nepal into some kind of perspective. It was such a busy, rich and overwhelming experience. I have not felt so far out of my depth since. On the first day of the camp, there was an annoying little voice in my head chanting, 'You can't do this, and you don't have to stay!' But I did." It is no surprise that culture shock can be severe. Nepali medical camps are an extreme experience for the newcomer.

Meanwhile, Eka Dev had gone on a tour of the far west, taking reports of the Bajhang and Bajura camps with him to give to the Regional Director of Health, who was very welcoming. He was particularly keen for ear and surgical camps, anywhere in the Far Western Region. "I will give you as much support as I can," he said. It seemed another group was doing some women's camps, though they were referring patients to other centres for major surgery, giving the patients money for that purpose.

Other team members did a small survey of ear disease in Pokhara schools. Pokhara had become a city and had good medical care with three large hospitals, one an Indian teaching hospital. One would expect very little untreated chronic ear disease there. Nevertheless 13 children were found with ear disease needing treatment, so a bus was arranged to take them from the city, a long day's journey into the hills to the next ear camp in May at Arughat, to the northwest of Kathmandu, where Mike Smith was operating.

Camps in May come with some risk. There can be devastating hail storms, and it is very hot. So this was another experiment! Three camps were planned. There was only a health centre, a small building, so the big INF marquee was borrowed and erected. The first camp was for gynaecology, followed by a joint ear and dental camp. The plan was to drive up the part hard-surfaced, part dry-weather (dusty) road, an eight-hour drive to cover the 80 miles. Arughat is on the main trekking route to Mt Manaslu. In 2008, it was said to have two lodges. By 2018, it had four hotels, charging £75 per night (ref Rome2Rio). Such is development. However, as so often, the best laid plans go astray, and the Maoists were still active. The road was blocked and there was a general strike.

Gynaecologist Sarah Caukwell walked across Kathmandu to see the sad sight of the former Royal Palace, now a museum but with the rooms where the massacre of most members of the royal family happened sealed off.

Sarah recalls: "Ellen was wondering how all the team members would get to Arughat. She considered a tourist bus with a permit, but none was available. So in typical fashion, she picked up the phone and within a few minutes had booked three helicopters for 6 am next morning." Later, the vehicles were able to get through. The health post was on a ridge, 20 minutes above the town. "The 25-minute helicopter ride was exhilarating, and all the town came out to greet us. There was a formal welcome, and we were given garlands of bougainvillea flowers. The marquee was used as a waiting and recovery area, but it was so hot! The hotel was nice, with a little garden and, as always, the food was rice with daal and vegetable curry. I'm still not keen on it."

Surgery went well, apart from one woman. She hadn't stayed after surgery for post-operative care, and was brought back three days later in a collapsed state. She had bled and was not fit for more surgery. Some team members gave their O positive blood but she still deteriorated. They attempted, as a last resort, to take her through the night to Kathmandu, but she died on the journey. After it was agreed on the phone, her body was returned to the village and was soon cremated, a grievous end for the family and the team, one of a tiny number of patients who had serious complications, among the 10,000 others who were safely treated.

Post-op gynaecology patients were cared for in the marquee. For the ear and dental camp, it was used for outpatients. It was up to 40°C and some of the team wanted to rest. However, true to the spirit of the old Shining Hospital, the show must go on—and it did! Despite the heat, an astonishing amount of work was achieved: 1,010 women were seen, with 111 operations; 789 ear clinic outpatients, with 92 for surgery; and the dentists extracted 579 teeth and did 91 fillings—not too much conservation of teeth there! These camps lasted eight days each.

At the ear camp there were British, Australian and Danish volunteers. Steve Broomfield, a surgeon from the UK wrote: 'The environment was unfamiliar, not least, dealing with the heat and insects in theatre! I was very conscious that the anaesthesia gave limited time for each operation, and that we could not afford to have any surgical complications. This camp had 3 surgeons, two experienced and myself, a senior trainee at the time. I had to learn fast and keep going!

However, Mike and Per Thomassen were very supportive and under their supervision I found the operative experience to be one of the highlights of the camp. On the last morning, all the patients who had undergone operations returned to have their wounds checked and bandages changed. This was an impressive sight. All patients were given detailed instructions on how to look after their ears, and a supply of ear drops, creams and dressings." Local paramedics were always involved, and clinic staff and patients were given contact numbers to reach the team in Pokhara if they had any problems.

Ellen's conclusion: "Never again in May. It was too hot, even in the hills. There was no breeze. The three teams were great, with no complaints. On the day we left Arughat, the heavens opened and torrential rain caused us to slide down the 'fair weather' road. Fortunately, no vehicles got stuck in the mud." This area would be near the epicentre of the 7.9 strength earthquake which struck in 2015. Many buildings were destroyed and many, many killed. Nepal is a tragic country. In every monsoon, when 200 inches of rain can fall in three months, there is destruction and death from flooding rivers and landslides on the steep deforested hillsides, often sweeping away half or even all of a village. The trekkers and visitors rarely see this side of life.

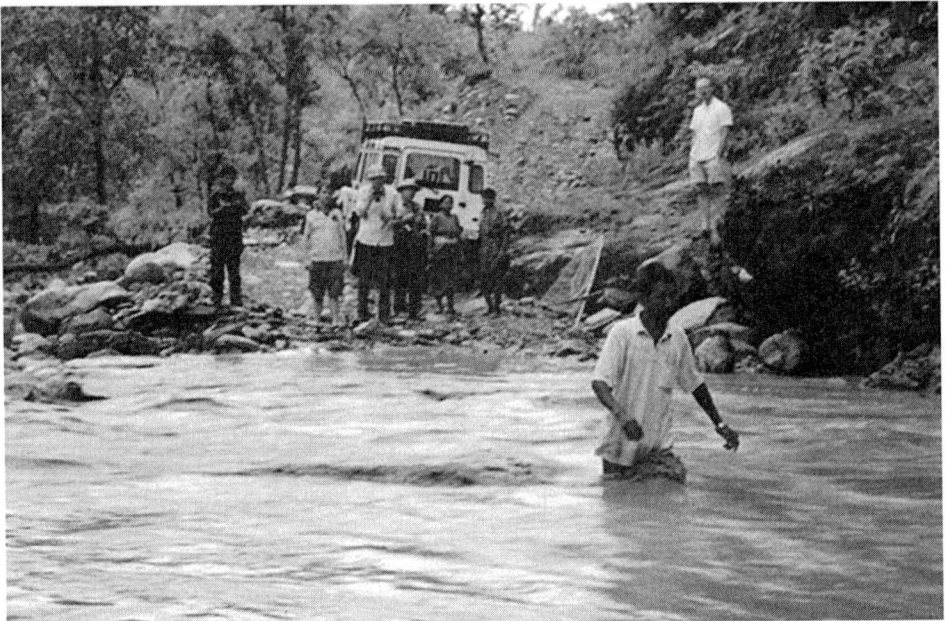

*River in flood near Awalching.*

# Chapter 19

## New Possibilities

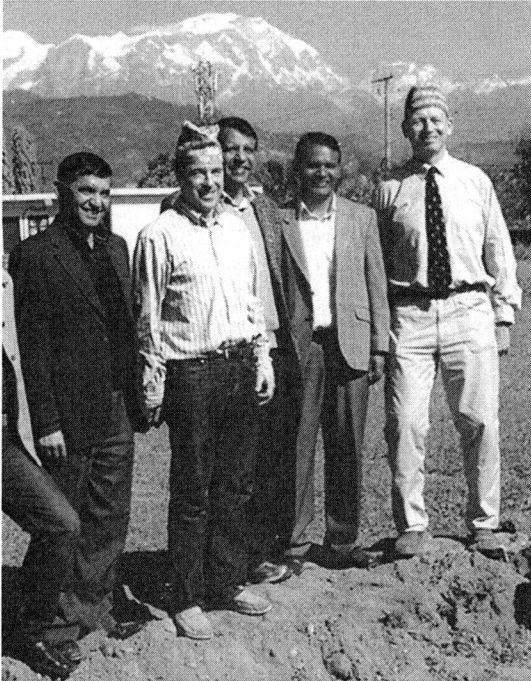

*Mission leaders: Prem Subedi, Deependra Gautam and Krishna Adhikari, with Lukas and Mike, lay the foundation stone for the ear centre.*

At about this time, new ideas were developing. For the first time, in a letter from Mike Smith to Ellen, a possibility was raised. Was it feasible to have an ear hospital in Pokhara? Others doubted it.

He now started looking for possible sites in western Nepal with sufficient infrastructure. He considered the government Western Regional Hospital where he had previously worked in Pokhara, but after discussing with some doctors working there it sounded unlikely to be a priority for the hospital at that time, although it would have been attractive to integrate with the government system. There was a central site in Pokhara where a private hospital had shut down. It was not quite right. He approached another hospital who said no. As he looked for vacant land, the Director of INF said, "Why not look at Green Pastures? There is plenty of land there." Indeed there was. Mike had worked there before and he knew the site well.

Green Pastures had moved on. As well as leprosy treatment, it had become a rehabilitation centre for people severely injured in the fighting or from accidents. There was land available and very suitable.

The planning work began—a lengthy process anywhere. The big question was how to fund it. INF had several sponsors for other established work but not for this. Lukas Eberle had enthusiastically worked with Mike in the ear camps, coming every couple of years. He had learned much from Mike to take back to his own practice in Brunnen, near Lake Lucerne, Switzerland. He had put funds into camps and was inspired to take the cause of ear camps to medical and other groups in Switzerland. When he heard about the plans, he offered to raise the entire sum needed to build the hospital, and a Swiss charity, SON, (Stiftung Ohrchirurgie Nepal) was formed, with support from medical teams in Lucerne and Zurich (where Lukas trained).

About the same time in 2010, Shirley Heywood began to run fistula camps. Having returned from Ethiopia with specialist training, she ran a series of one-week camps in Surkhet. Eka Dev did the advertising via local radio, inviting people to phone him to make an appointment.

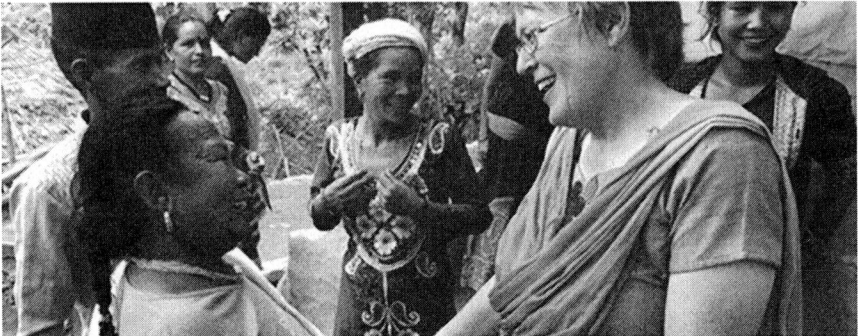

*Dr Shirley Heywood with one of her patients.*

The camps team travelled to Surkhet with necessary equipment and theatre staff. "I reckon we could have 50 patients next year," said Eka Dev as phone calls kept coming. So, they prepared for this possibility and borrowed the INF marquee for the patients to recover in. The camp lasted three weeks and 56 operations were performed.

Whilst home, Shirley met up with a retired urologist, Mike Bishop, a fistula specialist who travelled the world. He then came to Surkhet every year from 2011 to 2018, helping out (except 2017 when visas were refused). As the new government hospital in Surkhet was being built, it was possible for the post-op patients to recover in the foyer, avoiding the scenario of holding down a marquee as storms threatened to swamp it and blow it away! It meant relatives carrying patients 200 yards from the theatre. Two trusts came on board, the Talbot Trust and the Fistula Foundation, plus a small American Trust, Help for Our Sisters. They supplied instruments and general camp costs, allowing the training of nurses, and health promotion and awareness talks in all the districts in West, Mid-West, and Far West regions—a big task in these remote areas. Two-day training was carried out in all areas.

Meanwhile, camps continued. Ellen's sister had become ill, and Ellen made the decision to stay with her. Long before this time, the Nepali team was fully competent to organise camps and transport for the expatriate teams. The next camp was for gynaecology problems in Arghakhanchi, now with better roads, accessible from Pokhara. It was quieter than usual as another group had been there a year before and had given money for the women to go to their regional centre. Some went but felt scared and alone in a big town and returned home, then came back to this camp. However, at the end, considering the other groups now offering help to women, the camp leaders decided to reduce gynaecology camps to one a year and increase surgical camps. It is always real progress when others start taking over. The long-term objective must be for Nepal to be able to care for its own. Ellen wrote, "We realise that all medical camps are temporary but in the meantime they fill a gaping hole in the health system."

Both the ear and surgical camps were held in Baitadi, the district bordering the Indian Himalayan foothills. Some patients at the surgical camp were referred to Kathmandu, 530 miles away by road! The team was in a different health centre from the previous visit to Baitadi; it was held in a small town called Patan. Ellen's concern was for the Nepali team who would be away for five weeks. She knew that poor accommodation and food affected them too, and she was concerned for their welfare.

The ear camp had its usual large crowd of patients, with several returning to have their second ear operated on, having regained hearing in the first. A couple brought their son with cerebral palsy to have surgery. Fathers would walk for days bringing their children with discharging ears. 126 people had surgery, but the really busy people were the audiology team who did 550 hearing tests and fitted 240 hearing aids. One elderly couple returned their hearing aids. They couldn't stand the sound of each other's voice and preferred silence!

Jyoti Thapa, an experienced Nepali audiologist, working in the UK, returned to her homeland as a volunteer. She wrote an article for a Nepali newspaper about her experiences, including these observations: "All three of us audiologists were working in the same room, battling with the language barrier (even I needed help from the two nurses helping with translation, as not everyone understood my Kathmandu Nepali), while trying to ignore the ebb and flow of ambient noise, such as phones ringing, people shouting and babies crying. It was by no means an ideal way to perform hearing tests, but we could not insist on soundproof booths! We performed tests on ourselves to find and apply correction factors. We rapidly learned to work the best we could within the existing conditions. Our task alternated between being frustrating, fatiguing and funny. Most patients seemed to be totally baffled by the concept of sounds being delivered by the headphones to each ear separately. We taught them to raise an arm when they heard a sound in the headphone. Some locals pointed out, half-jokingly, that this looked like the Maoist army salute! We tested all ages, from a 94-year-old grannie to a one-year-old child. Some were smartly dressed, others turned up in clothes that were falling to bits with wear and grime. There were teachers, farmers and labourers. What struck me hard was the harshness of life and malnourishment that made some 17-year-olds look like 10, and some 40-year-olds look like 60. There were precious snippets of joy, such as when a woman fitted with a hearing aid cried as she heard sounds for the first time in many years. We also experienced great sadness when we saw children as old as 10 with a profound hearing loss, whose parents brought them to the camp with the hope that surgery or hearing aids could do something for them. I personally found it heart-wrenching to explain that their level of hearing loss was unlikely to benefit from aids and in any case, they were past the age of spoken language acquisition. The best we could advise was to enroll in a school for the deaf, to gain some literacy and learn Nepali sign language. We advised them not to spend money on medicines. Some had been prescribed medicines elsewhere, supposedly to cure nerve deafness. I personally was very touched by the level of commitment I saw in the different individuals who had come together for the camp. Being Nepali I could justify the visit as an opportunity to make my annual visit to family. At the best, these people, who paid their own fares and expenses, and took annual leave to attend, might receive a smile or a coy 'Thank you' in return for all their effort. At the worst, their work might be dismissed as a conscience-washing-exercise, (although writing a cheque to a charity would be infinitely easier!). I saw it as a sort of internationalism whereby people, for whatever reason, came to help total strangers."

Jo, a young anaesthetist on the team, wrote frankly in his report: "Misconceptions encountered by a trainee: 'They're a bunch of Christian do-gooders'; but I found the expatriate team was of mixed ethnic, gender and religious backgrounds and I certainly did not notice any preaching or religious recruiting. The overriding feeling was of being there to do the best job possible. The second misconception: 'You'll be performing procedures to standards which would be unacceptably low in the UK' was also rapidly disproved; we had four ENT specialists and two anaesthetists, including Charlie Collins, who was in his 17th year of camps. As I worked with such experienced colleagues, my own technique improved as camp progressed."

The general surgeons were also overrun. Ultrasound was so useful for diagnosis, and 216 people were assessed. Many had major surgery, two, fortunately, arriving in time for urgent life-saving operations—a week later there would have been no-one to treat them.

It was the desire of the Nepali team to expand into new territories. The spring camps of 2011 were to be held in Gokuleshwar, Darchula District. You could go no further to the west in Nepal. This area bordered both India and Tibet, its highest point being Api Himal at 23,400 ft. To its south was Bajura; to its east was Bajhang. It has a population of 133,000. Most interesting is the revelation that in the 2011 census, 6,500 of its people worked abroad, mainly as night watchmen, security guards and labourers in India or the Middle East. That must surely be true of all these remote areas where food is scarce. Unfortunately, one side effect of this is that HIV infection, leading to AIDs is sometimes brought into the remote areas when workers return to their families. There is a trade route to Tibet and woven goods are exchanged. Yak butter (ghee) is traded by those who live on the high ground. This camp was going to be challenging, not least, getting there. Back-to-back seven to eight-day camps were planned for February, a cold time at altitude but dry with sunny days. It was not surprising that the number of women was fewer than in most camps. Agricultural work is demanding, carrying water and foraging for grass for the buffaloes. Nevertheless, 678 people did come for examination, and 62 of them had operations. A major issue was infertility and, where possible, the man was tested. There was a high rate of male infertility.

This gynaecology camp was followed by an ear camp led by Mike. It was busy, and to meet the need, work started at 8 am and finished at 10 pm. Mike had stamina and everyone else sought to keep up! 147 operations were performed, but some patients had to be turned away. Audiology was busier than ever. If the camp was barely manageable for the surgical team, it was hard on the patients too. Only a certain number of 'tickets' were given out each day, and people waited two nights out in the open on a stone courtyard under the eaves of the hospital, sleeping under thin blankets in rows. They were very patient as they quietly waited for help. The team were shocked to see this as they arrived each morning. We hoped that, in this crowd of needy humanity, each individual would feel they were important and cared for. Ellen was brilliant at this.

A mother brought her four boys, all profoundly deaf. They were now too old to have cochlear implants. Another man heard about camp from a returning student and walked two days to get there. Both ears were discharging. One was operated on, and he would return to another camp for the other ear. This was a normal practice. It was delightful for all when a patient returned saying, "I can hear. Please do the other one." Occasionally, when a patient had very severe, even life-threatening infection in both ears, the team would operate on one ear at the beginning of the camp and, if all was well, do the other ear a few days later.

There were many disturbing situations. One man wanted to take his wife home early, the morning after surgery. "We only live one hour's walk away. She is the only one who is able to get the buffalo out without being attacked." A small, mentally disabled boy came with both his ears cut off. The team was told, "His ears were bitten off by the dog." A very sad situation and it was impossible to know what had actually happened. Another boy had a huge haemangioma (benign blood vessel tumour) filling his mouth, and forcing his tongue out, far too risky to operate at the camp. They could only advise, offer financial help and hope he would get treatment in a good centre in Kathmandu or India. It is impossible for local families to know what to do in such a distressing situation and how to access good, safe, economic care.

The hospital assigned five local paramedical staff to work with the team, and to be taught as they worked, a very welcome opportunity. Seeing so much complicated pathology in this camp spurred Mike on to draw up plans for his vision of an ear hospital and training centre.

It was not all work, Mike and colleagues, surgeons John and Tristram, and audiologist Charlotte, managed to get a rare flight up to Dolpa and trek to the beautiful Phoksundo lake. It was February, so there was plenty of snow on the ground and most of the tiny villages were empty, as the people had gone down to lower altitudes with their animals for the winter. They saw snow leopard tracks, and flocks of the elusive Himalayan blue sheep. Sadly, although their young guide claimed to have seen them, they did not find any yeti.

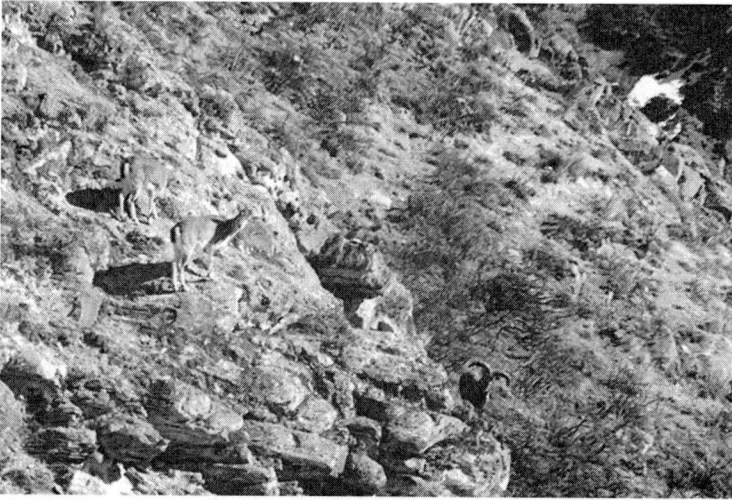

*'Himalayan Blue sheep', well camouflaged against the rocks, near Phoksundo.*

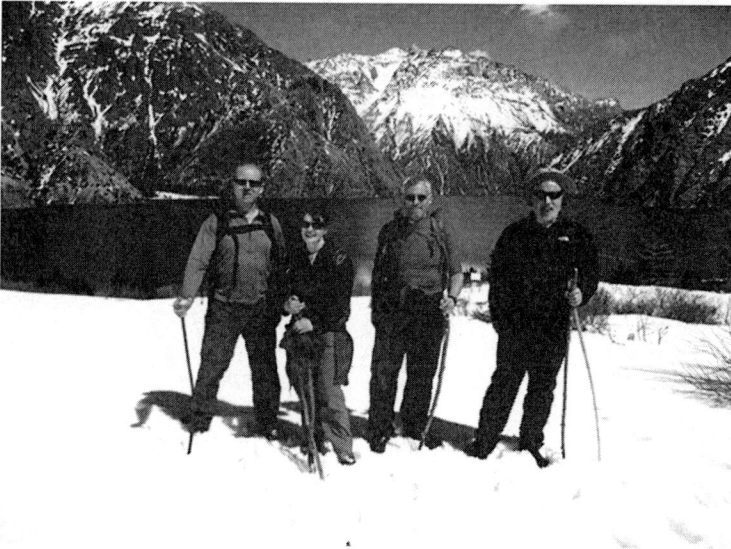

*Mike, Charlotte, John and Tristram at Phoksundo lake.*

Standing back, looking at those numbers, the volume of work was amazing. Mercifully, in all the camp reports received, with thousands of operations in each specialty being done under basic conditions, only one fatality has been recorded, except in patients with terminal illness.

Follow-up of ear patients was difficult. Over the years, only 10% of those that had surgery were seen again, despite many efforts to revisit and recall them. Nonetheless, analysis of the data and comparison with results for camps with higher follow-up rates showed amazingly good outcomes.

The time back in Scotland had been hard for Ellen. She, with help from her other sister, had nursed her sister, Rena, for some months before she died. It was very sad. Ellen reflected: "Life is now beginning to settle into a routine and my thoughts are turning to other things." That included returning to Nepal for the gynaecology camp in Dailekh. That was immediately followed by the ear and surgical camps in equally remote Mangalsen, principal town in Achham, with 32,000 people. "The roads were much better than in 2006, but the journey still took 14 hours from Nepalganj (after flying from Kathmandu). The return journey was easier as we spent a night on the way. We were made very welcome."

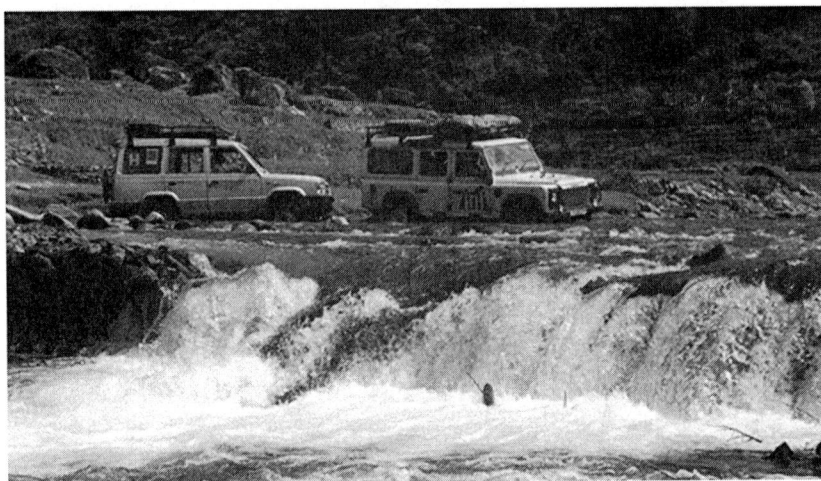

*One of many obstacles on the fair-weather road.*

Dr Ian Ferrer, who attended many camps as a GP and who, with his wife, Claire, had previously worked with INF for some years, recalled that the hotel was dreadful: "It had to be fumigated with toxic spray from the bazaar. It nearly did for me too. Generally, I was happy as long as the food, usually daal bhat, was good." He always took a camping mat and a sheet or sleeping bag. "Sometimes, in health centres, we had to sleep on the stone floor, but hotels could be good. I was prepared. The operating suite was available, as was water. We needed our generators, as the local electricity supply was inadequate."

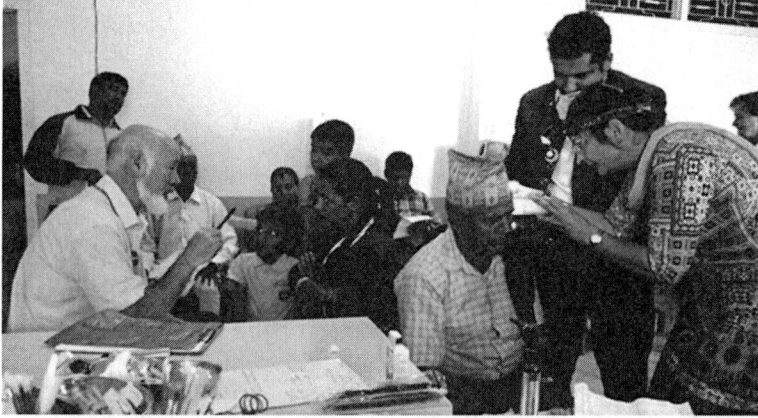

*Ian and Claire Ferrer on a general medical camp.*

The ear camp had four surgeons, including a Nepali ENT surgeon, from Kathmandu (Dr Kashi Raj Gyawali), Lukas Eberle, and another regular, Derek Skinner from the UK. Derek was famous for being able to power nap anywhere, any time. Several times he was found asleep, sitting upright on a small surgeon's stool, but not while operating! Lukas brought several Swiss and German specialists including the dedicated Walter, and his colleague Sonja. They were like machines, fitting digital hearing aids with the computer, making ear moulds, taking immense care and pride in how they helped each patient. Walter kept his age a close secret, but he attended several camps, and must have been in his 80s. Hearing aids had moved on. Previously donated aids were all analogue, (the types with a volume dial, which were often quite large). Now they were receiving digital aids from several countries. These all required a computer, correct software, and wire leads. They gave much better hearing, could be adjusted more accurately to match the patient's needs, and were smaller and neater, but all these requirements made for more preparation and more equipment. Walter could be found late into the evening, hunched over his computer, programming aids for the next day.

They were all kept busy as the numbers attending seemed to be ever increasing. 1,367 people were seen in outpatients, with 141 operations. This 10% figure seemed to repeat in most ear camps. The Nepali trainee commented to Ellen, "I have never worked with such an experienced surgeon as Mike and he

167

is so humble. Tell me what motivates him." So, Ellen did! The feature at this camp was that 37 patients returned for a second ear operation. A 12-year-old girl had pus running from a fistula behind her ear. The dead bone was removed and the ear reconstructed. Many, needing less urgent myringoplasty had to be turned away.

Even before the general surgeons had arrived for the next camp in Achham, hundreds of patients had registered. Many patients were assessed and, where appropriate, treated by the GP.

One woman had a massive 10 kg ovarian cyst removed [more than 3 times the size of an average Nepali new born baby!]. 12 patients whose kidney stones were removed needed great care to ensure the blood supply to the kidney was not damaged. Such complex surgery also creates an added demand on the anaesthetist, with less than ideal equipment. A man with bladder cancer was referred to Kathmandu, which may have seemed like the end of the earth to this village man. Altogether, 1147 patients were seen and treated, 334 had ultrasound scans, 107 had operations and 67 had haemorrhoids banded. This all occurred in 6.5 days!

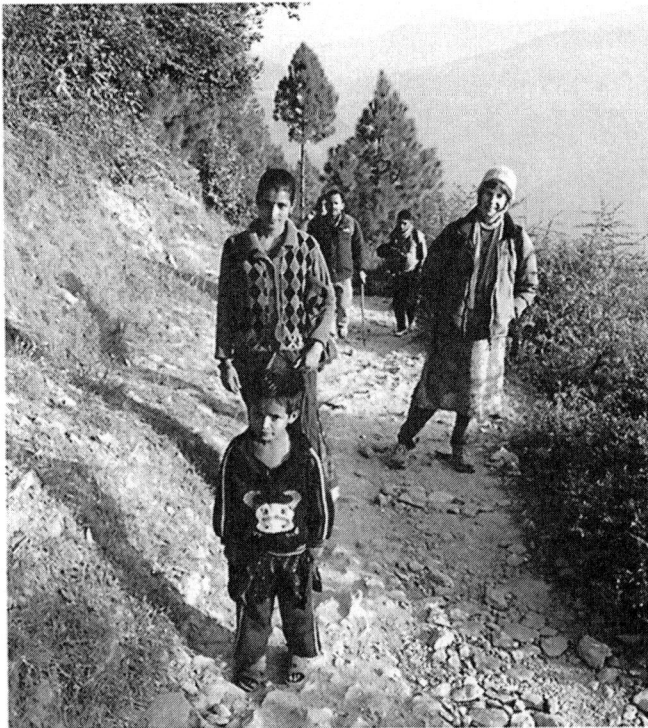

*A young patient and her mum walk to the hospital, with Jo Bissett.*

168

Ian remembers: "There was a 30-minute walk from our 'hotel' to the hospital. The people were extremely trusting and welcoming. I was especially touched when I met a seven-year-old girl walking up to the hospital for her operation, and she walked the rest of the way happily holding my hand, with her mother dragging behind.

"Training was also a feature of this camp. A local health worker learnt how to administer and monitor a spinal anaesthetic, as well as monitoring general anaesthesia. Ward nurses learnt how to care for post-operative patients and look after drains and catheters. Visiting surgeon, Dr Bhoj Raj Neupane, taught how conditions could be managed in Nepal, while he himself was up-skilled in surgical techniques.

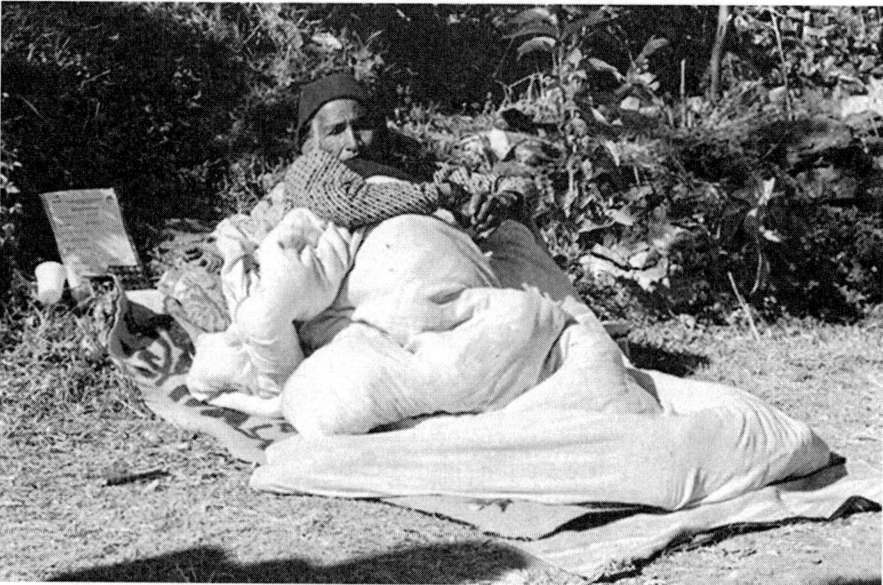

*A patient recovers from surgery, sitting in the sunshine, with medical chart and medicines at hand!*

"The camp was a great success, and the Chief District Officer thanked each of us individually at the end of camp. The extra travelling time reduced operating time, but we certainly made a difference for a big group of people."

# Chapter 20

## 2012

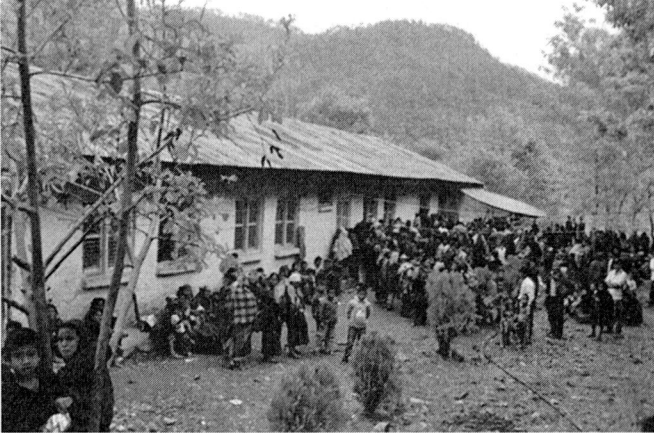

*Crowds gather at a district hospital, waiting for a check-up.*

Ellen, writing home, tells the story of this year: "Thank you for your prayers and support. Our camps in Kolti and Bajura went very well. The two teams accepted the tough conditions in Kolti without complaint. They worked long hours, the ear team working from 9 am to 2 am some days! Time for a couple of hours sleep, then start again!" Having come so far, with the expertise and equipment, and seeing the needs among people who would have little other chance of treatment, all agreed that they were there to work and help as many as possible. It was often possible to have a free afternoon at the end of the camp to take a walk-up a nearby hill or explore the bazaar. The visitors loved seeing the villages, the people at work in the fields and farms, and the beautiful scenery.

"Following on from the ear camp, we had three gynaecologists and some operations lasted a long time, up to four hours. We had women with no uterus and others with two (bicornuate). Another woman, who had gone from hospital to hospital for infertility treatment, was finally wrongly told that she had no uterus. She came to us, and a pregnancy test showed she was three months pregnant! She couldn't believe her ears, then saw the baby's heart beat on a scan. WOW!

"A woman came with a fistula, leaking urine since giving birth two years earlier. She had sought help elsewhere and spent £2,000 on ineffective treatment (her earnings were £40 per month). Our visiting Australian gynaecologist specialised in fistulas and spent four hours operating on her. Because another camp followed on, we were able to keep a catheter in for a fortnight to allow healing. The need for a fistula centre was increasingly clear.

"A sad woman stood at the table, a piece of paper crumpled in her hand. Her husband had gone to India to earn money and did not return for ten years. They had two children, then the husband died. It was then that she found out he had AIDS and she and the second child were now HIV+.

"As the ear camp was drawing to a close, and final operating lists were prepared, a seriously ill woman living 15 minutes away turned up with pus flowing from her ear. She couldn't come earlier as she had work to do! Immediate operation was impossible due to the acute infection and we gave her 24 hours of IV antibiotics. Then, having discharged the rest of the patients, she had a three-hour operation. Mike wanted to do a minor procedure on her other ear, to prevent it becoming as bad. The family refused. 'She has to care for the children. She has work to do.' There is fear that healing may be compromised. She was advised to come to our next ear camp for the second ear, but I doubt she will be allowed. Can she afford to travel? These people have a hand-to-mouth existence.

"Travelling to Burtibang nine hours by jeep for the November gynaecology and ear camp was likened to a motocross/hill climb that people pay good money to take part in! We had the sport for free! The road was rough for seven hours but better than the two-day walk when we came 15 years ago. The locals were appreciative of the camps. Patients came to say, 'Thank you.' It was very moving for one member of the staff, who had never experienced this before and cried. INF members had worked for years in this small town of 7,000, though not now. They were fondly remembered by name.

"The government now requires all medical camps to be approved by the health ministry, but as we had worked through the years with the minister, approval was given. As usual these days, more people needed help than we had time to treat, but Burtibang is not as remote as the areas in the far west."

Sandra Chinnery added her story of Burtibang: "'How many children do you have?' I asked. 'Five. Four girls and a boy,' the lady replied. 'Was the fifth one a boy?' I asked. 'Yes. Life was terrible before that. My husband beat me after

171

each baby was born, pulling me by my hair and treating me cruelly. After our fourth baby girl was born, he married another wife. We lived in one house together. A little while later, our son was born. Since then, my husband shows me more respect.'"

The team worked in the local school buildings. "It was a blessing being there, passing on medicines, hope, and love." Sandra wrote of a tragedy. "Five young Australians had spent time on holiday in Surkhet after Christmas. On their journey in a minibus returning to Kathmandu, their vehicle was hit by a bus cutting a corner. Neer, asleep in the back, never woke up again. The others were seriously injured."

Mike was heading up his 40th camp. It was his wife Fiona's first camp. For her, the experience was wonderful, worthwhile, challenging and fun. Fiona wrote an overview: "Even though we had lived and worked in Nepal, this was my first camp. It turned out to be a huge adventure but also an enormous privilege. In late November, we had packed up over 100 kgs of baggage, thanks to Air India's generous allowance, including hundreds of hats knitted by friends for the patients. We met up with some members of the 15-strong team at Heathrow; others came direct to Nepal from Australia and New Zealand. Mike always tried to meet all the UK team members at Heathrow airport in London and utilise everyone's baggage allowance to take donated medical items with them. There was always much repacking to transport as much as possible. This could be quite stressful, but only once in 50 journeys did we have to pay excess baggage, thanks to a lot of careful preplanning." This time he had Fiona to help.

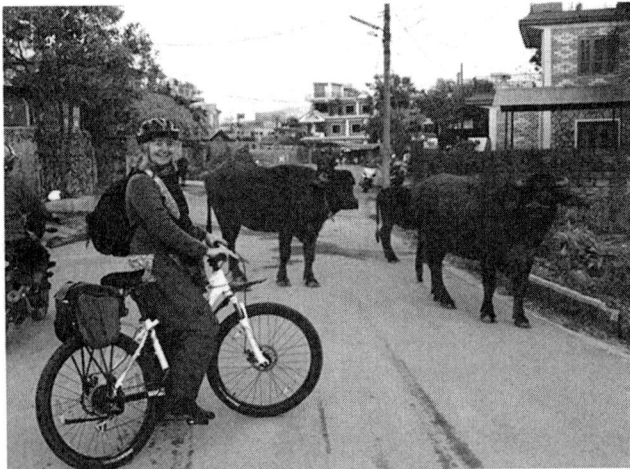

*Fiona dodges the buffaloes, to go shopping in Pokhara.*

"Far too excited to sleep, we enjoyed the majesty of the Himalayas as we flew the two hours from Delhi to Kathmandu. We found our minibus and were launched into the melee of traffic, holding onto our seats as we wove in and out of numerous motorbikes, trucks, and errant taxis. Our destination was the Summit hotel perched above the smog of the city, where we were able to catch our breath and meet up with the rest of the team. Next day we flew in a 30-seat plane to Pokhara, gasping at the beauty of the Annapurnas, Dhaulagiri, Hiunchuli and Ganesh Himal—all a trekkers paradise. The final part of the journey was an eight-hour, off-road, nail-biting Land Rover trip to Burtibang, crossing three bridges over rivers (described by Mike as exhilarating!). Our hotel was good, with omelette and tea for breakfast, samosas and onion bhajis at the hospital for lunch and daal bhat plus pieces of the chickens we had walked past in the morning, for the evening meal!

"On arrival, we had a look at the hospital where we would work for nine days. It was half built, with no glass in the windows and some cement not quite set, so it was damp. The wind whistled through the gaps, and we all donned warm clothes under our scrubs. We saw about 200 patients a day, 152 had surgery, and the audiology team fitted 200 hearing aids, working from 9 am – 7 pm... legendary! The camp worked like clockwork, a tribute to Ellen, Mike, and the Nepali team, working with a well-tried formula. A young couple brought their three-year-old son with Down's syndrome. He was unable to walk and had no speech. They were hoping for a miracle cure. Ellen sat quietly with them and explained that cure was not possible, but that such children are loving and respond to love, it would not help to travel around looking for expensive treatments. Another boy of about eight years came with an itchy, infected ear. Everyone gathered to see what was removed – three dead baby cockroaches!"

Ellen recalled some of the patients: "A man brought his two sisters. Both had suddenly become deaf, one 21 years ago, the other five years back. They thought a hearing test was a waste of time and went home but came back next day. They had the test, and both were suitable for hearing aids. They were excited to hear for the first time in years and shouted, 'I can hear. I can hear.'

"Separate from the camp, the hospital sister asked me to help her with dressings for a man badly burned when a kerosene stove blew up. I could see he would be in even greater agony when we changed the dressings, so I asked our anaesthetist to give him sedation. Soon afterwards, we heard a helicopter arrive. It had been sent by this man's brother to take him to Kathmandu. The man was a Maoist and his brother was a government minister.

"If ever I had a doubt about the vision for an ear hospital in Pokhara, which I didn't, this visit to Burtibang convinced me that this was the right way forward. People who needed hospitalisation for intensive treatment included a woman with a facial paralysis following a badly infected ear as a child, and children needing cochlear implants with follow-up speech therapy. So many needed surgery and hearing aids."

At the end of the camp, Mike wrote home, giving an update on the progress of the ear hospital: "The plans are complete. The INF team in Nepal have engineers and a project manager. We go to tender soon. The vision is to alleviate lifelong suffering and sometimes life-threatening ear disease, which can cut people off from communication, education and development, especially the poor.

"It will be a centre for referral from camps. It will train audiologists and specialist doctors. Core services should be self-funding as those who can pay for their treatment will pay some charge. A charity, Ear Aid Nepal has been set up in the UK to help fund the poor and provide teaching materials, equipment and information for potential volunteers and trainers. Dr Lukas Eberle has worked with us many times and his Swiss charity has already raised £400,000 of the £1 million needed, and other funds have come through INF. We have also approached the German government."

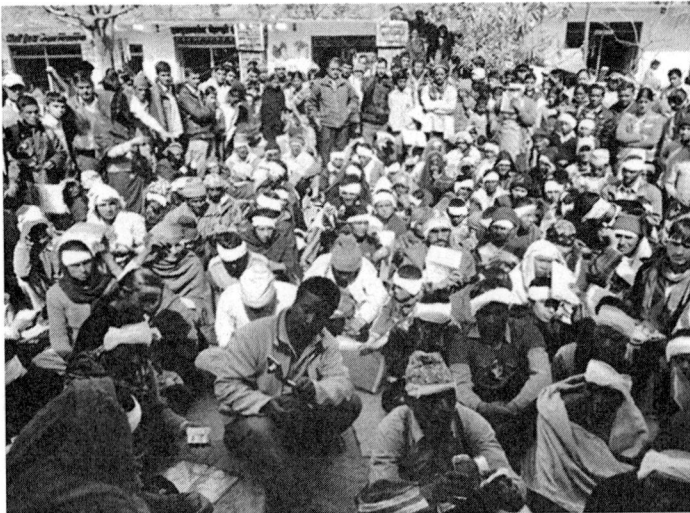

*Ear camp patients get their post-op medicines, instructions and contact details.*

# Chapter 21

## A Nepali Perspective

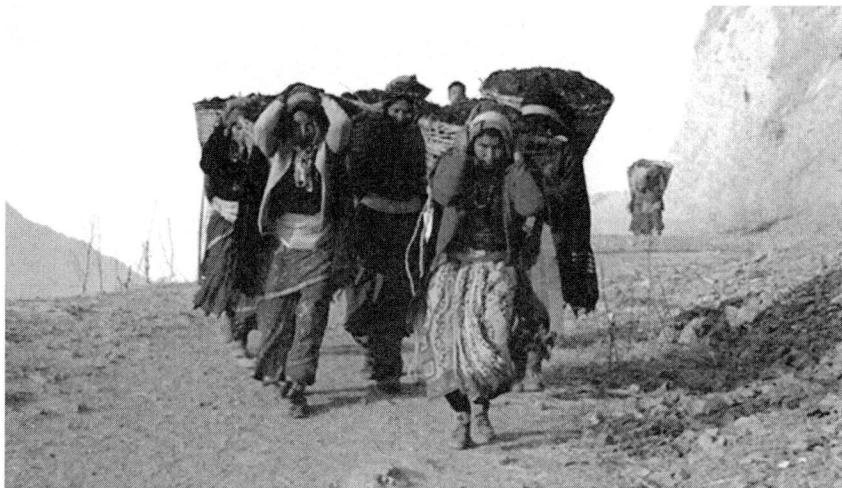

*Women's lives are harsh, carrying fodder, water, firewood every day.*

Much had changed in Nepal. The new Republic was finding its feet. There was an urgent need to draw up a new constitution and this was to become a long-running saga of disagreements. Finally, it was produced in September 2015. Prior to this, the new republic had begun to indicate to Non-Governmental Organisations (NGOs) that change was afoot. Refusal to renew work visas for those expatriates working in Nepal for more than ten years gave hints of more restrictions to come. The underlying plan seemed to be that NGO projects should be put into the hands of Nepalis. INF was already beginning to do that, making trained Nepalis heads of projects. Effectively, that had happened long ago in INF camps. Eka Dev, supported by his team, were doing all the planning, liaison with officials and local authorities, followed by preparation and transport of equipment and personnel, and site preparation. Ellen and Mike found and liaised with the visiting specialists.

The first two camps of 2013 were held back-to-back in distant Bajhang. One of the team for the first camp was a young Nepali, Arpan, from a Pokhara family, soon to be studying medicine in China. The plan was to allow him to experience the issues faced by a doctor sent by the Nepali government to a rural location and to see the possibilities of bringing medical help to poor and remote communities. It was felt that this experience would be a good backcloth to his medical training. He takes up the story:

"I was invited to join a surgical camp in the far west of Nepal, at a place called Bajhang, early in 2013. It was a huge opportunity because it was unusual for non-INF Nepali staff to join in on the surgical camps and I was given the chance to experience camp as a volunteer. I am very grateful to the people who made it happen.

"I had just been accepted at the Sun Yat-Sen University of Medical Science in China for the class of September 2013, so this surgical camp was a boost-up for me and my journey towards the field of medicine. I was really excited.

"It was a gruesome three-day drive to the village in Bajhang. We had one big truck full of equipment and three INF Land Rovers for the advance party. We drove 10–12 hours each day and arrived exhausted but with great enthusiasm. The people I went with were the nicest people. They always included me, so I never felt left out.

"The hotel we were staying in had three storeys and tiny rooms. Breakfast of omelette and bread was taken in the sun on the roof. I shared my room with another member of staff. We were served typical Nepalese dishes every day. Fourteen of us Nepalese spent the whole day unloading and setting up the district hospital. We cleaned it and set it up for the two weeks of surgical and then ear camps. The first group of foreign doctors and nurses arrived the next day to a well-equipped hospital ready for work.

"From the hotel to the hospital took about 10 minutes involving a 200-metre suspension bridge over the Seti River. For the first few days, I worked with the GPs, helping them with translation and communication with the patients. The doctors and the foreign volunteers were all kind and let me experience every place in the hospital where I could learn and get inspired. The two nurses who came for that trip were so helpful; they helped me learn a few techniques and shared a lot of knowledge.

"The one thing that was difficult for me, even though I am a Nepali, was the food! It was tasty, but half the time we didn't know what we were eating! I remember the second day of the surgeries. For lunch we had traditional Nepali thali with mutton. I had eaten mutton before, but this one tasted 'non-muttony'.

176

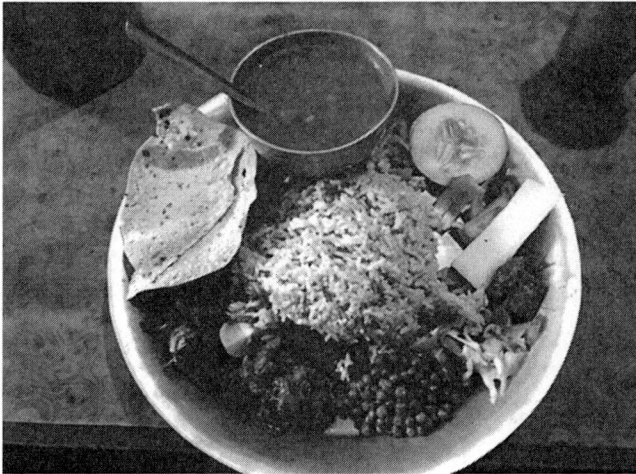

*A rather better plate of Nepali daal bhat than usually available on a camp!*

Being polite guests, the surgeons and those who were on lunch break ate it with delight. It tasted good, until all of us suffered diarrhoea that night. I will not forget the next day when I went to work but had to give up half-way through as I felt so weak. But what else could you ask for but a bunch of great doctors around you when you are sick! We all got back to work on medication. We were too busy, and our minds were fixed on helping as many people as possible. This mindset helped us get through all the difficulties and inconveniences.

"Overall, my experiences there were unforgettable. I am to this very day thankful to INF and Ellen (I admire her heart) for making it possible for me to attend the Bajhang camp, which encouraged me to get to this stage. I am a medical intern in one of the best hospitals in South China now. I will be finished in a few months and I am looking forward to attending my next camp as a doctor."

In June 2019, Arpan graduated from his medical school in Guangzhou, China, as a doctor, and returned to Nepal to become registered there.

Arpan was not alone in his experience of illness at that camp. Food poisoning affected 15 of the 17-expatriate staff. Two needed IV drips. They struggled on and got through the work. Those present will remember it for a long time, also for multiple mishaps with vehicles. Two of the vehicles each had two punctures. Two surgical cases will also be remembered. A boy was found to have a staghorn stone in his kidney. Fortunately, the surgeon specialised in urology and was able to remove it safely. It required the boy to stay on the ward, then in a local hotel, until the end of the second camp. Another boy of 11 had been to various centres with abdominal pain, with no improvement. The surgeon suggested an ultrasound, which showed gallstones, and these were removed. A father brought his daughter who seemed to be unable to hear or respond to anybody. The surgeon examined her but found no cause. Ellen recognised the cause! "She has an evil spirit." "You don't believe that do you?" replied the surgeon. Ellen and others prayed for her. She quickly returned to normal, and they went home happy. These events are beyond our Western concepts but very real in many places.

The ear camp followed on. A trainee ENT surgeon from Liverpool wrote his impressions. He, with others, was delayed in Kathmandu by a strike. All doctors new to Nepal had to register with the Nepal Medical Council, at a cost of $80 and often an extra day spent in offices, on arrival. The strike delayed this by a day, so they arrived in Nepalganj late. After the 16-hour road trip, he found himself in the same hotel where Arpan had stayed. "It was very basic, with a very cold shower outside. Breakfast, an omelette, on the roof in the sun was wonderful. At the end of a long day, the daal bhat was welcome, as were the samosas at lunch time. The hospital was usually staffed by one doctor, who had to cope with everything that came. The everyday hardships these people endured were painfully obvious. The days were long and demanding, but as a trainee ENT surgeon, being exposed to a vast amount of ear disease and operating on difficult chronic ear problems was something I relished, and it made up for the long hours and the fatigue I felt. Most rewarding was the utmost gratitude of the patients. It left me with a sense of achievement that I had been able to help desperately needy people."

The three audiologists were also stretched, not least by the ambient noise levels (55 decibels), the wide range of ear moulds they had to fit and various types of used hearing aids. Senior audiologist, Joy wrote: "A family were all a-chatter when they realised that Auntie Manahra's new hearing aid enabled her to understand them talking normally for the first time in many years, when they arrived off the night bus. A middle-aged man, Sayar, of very sober demeanour, chose a smiley face icon to express his pleasure at receiving an aid. The mother of a 10-year-old with cerebral palsy and severe hearing loss was so pleased to see him smile and turn to her voice."

The autumn gynaecology camp was held in Pyuthan, remote, but one of the more comfortable camps, where hot showers were available! Two Nepali trainee specialists joined the camp to gain experience and learn good technique. They saw so many more operations than ever before in a short time. It wasn't as busy as usual, coinciding with the vital rice harvest, which took priority. It did mean more time for teaching. Then Dr KC Arun, a consultant ENT surgeon from Kathmandu joined the ear camp that followed on.

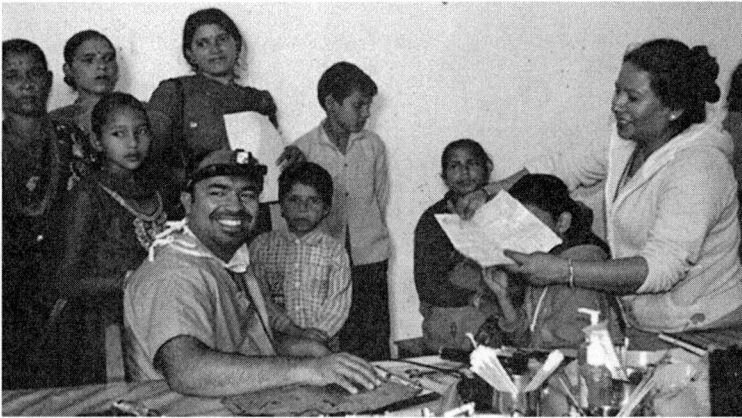

*Dr Arun joins an ear camp in Pyuthan in 2014.*

It was often difficult to recruit Nepali doctors as volunteers to attend camps. The uncertainty of food, travel and accommodation and leaving their regular practice and families was off-putting for them. They were usually subsidised, to encourage them to attend. In time, it became easier and more doctors did attend and benefitted by seeing new techniques, meeting colleagues and helping their own people. They had pressures unknown to the visiting volunteers, who only came for a short time. This was another reason why Mike felt that a base hospital providing high-quality care in Pokhara would be a good way to pass on skills.

There was a gap before the ear camp, as elections were being held in November, and the mood can be lively. The decision to hold the ear camp at Green Pastures hospital in Pokhara, in the rehabilitation centre and a marquee was a good way of advertising that an Ear Centre was being planned for that site. Indeed, building was almost ready to start, having obtained all necessary permissions. Lukas Eberle had brought a team of doctors from Switzerland to join in the camp and see the site and plans which they had generously funded.

"We wondered if patients would travel. In fact, there were hundreds, from all over the western half of Nepal and some from the east. When we asked them why they had travelled so far, they replied, 'We trust you. Your service is good.'

Some had had surgery at previous camps and had come for follow-up or surgery on the other ear. A depressed young man with no external ears, and deafness, had a bone conducting hearing aid fitted, and could now hear. He had a big smile. A 19-year-old student, Susmita, hoping to be a doctor, said that eight years ago she had a severe ear infection and Mike had saved her from meningitis. She now had a perforation in the other ear and was happy to see Mike again, even though she had travelled to Kathmandu and seen other doctors.

"Nam was a 27-year-old man from Pokhara. He was born deaf but could lip read. He came from a fairly poor family, his mother was a teacher, and his sister, who had been affected by polio, was a nurse, but his father, who had been a low-grade government worker, had died. In spite of Nam's huge disability, he was in his fourth year of electronic engineering training. He said he had been given a hearing aid years ago, with little benefit, so he stopped using it. Then he had surgery, but still could not hear. Today at the camp he had two new hearing aids fitted. When they were switched on, he could hear better for the first time in his life.

"The nine days saw an enormous volume of work. This confirmed the rightness of the decision to site the ear hospital here. When we told the patients this news on the last day when many were gathered for their post-operative dressings, they burst into applause."

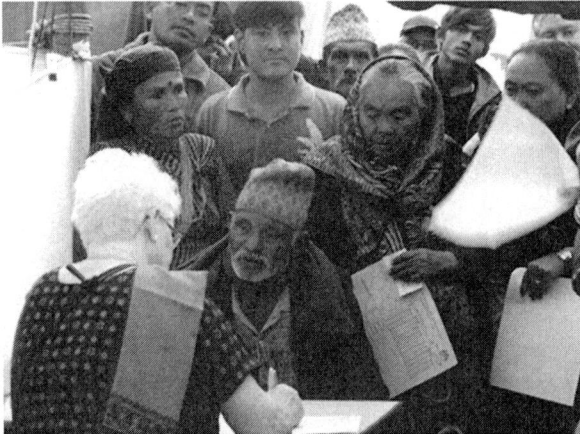

*Sister Ellen registers new patients and takes their medcal history in the tent at Green Pastures Hospital.*

At the end, the foundation stone was laid. Senior Nepali staff were very positive about the hospital. Mike Smith shared how the vision for the hospital began in a dream. "A boy with ear problems appeared in the dream and asked, 'Who will care for me when you are all gone?'" As Mike shared his heart with the assembled company, you could hear a pin drop. Now, three years later, his dream was being fulfilled. Lukas, through tremendous hard work, was on course to raise sufficient funds from Switzerland for the building. Amazingly, a German agency had also prioritised the ear centre for funding but was awaiting final approval. Then, due to a bureaucratic slip up in Germany, the final deadline had been missed. Astonishingly, those responsible were so sorry that they said "Draft a new application, including running costs for three years, and submit it for next year". According to Mike: "They were as good as their word, and it was successful. No donors pay hospital running costs! We could not believe it. This would give a good opportunity to get started well." Thomas Meier, an INF engineer, was an important intermediary with the German agency and also with SON—they much preferred dealing with a native German speaker who knew his way around their systems.

Ellen, waiting for hip surgery and with her polymyalgia improving, was delighted to be there in Pokhara for the laying of the stone, at what was to be called the 'Ear Hospital and Training Centre'. Near the end of the camp, Ellen's stiffness and pain suddenly returned. She was very unwell and unable to get out of bed. Fortunately, she had brought a nurse friend from home and after treatment from one of the anaesthetists she improved and, with help and support, continued to assist the work and then travel home.

The camps phase of her life had finally come to an end, and new things lay ahead. Camps themselves were also becoming difficult to run. There were many restrictions and delays in obtaining work visas and medical registration. Whilst it was understandable that specialists should be checked by the medical authorities, the system was very slow and cumbersome. It was becoming unrealistic to bring in volunteers. Ellen had been present at over 100 camps and had set up and trained her very able Nepali team. They had a truck which took 1,500kg of equipment to each camp - operating tables, oxygen concentrators, an oxygen cylinder, generator and fuel, plus the instruments, drapes, and gowns.

In addition to Ellen's extraordinary achievements as a visionary and instigator, she was the manager, trouble shooter, encourager and a remarkable and deeply compassionate nurse. It was so appropriate that her last camp was at Green Pastures, the place where she had spent many early years working with patients affected by leprosy.

It was Ellen who noticed, 20 years earlier, that almost all patients coming to the Western Regional Hospital did so by accessing a local bus route. She thought of those who could not reach a road or were far from a specialist hospital. Whilst it was hopelessly unrealistic to 'plant' clinics in all the districts of western Nepal, maybe something useful could be achieved by camps.

She and Mike devised a plan, the story of which has been told in these pages.

For the next 20 years, Ellen was present at almost all camps. 100,000 people attended those camps, each one given personal care by the team, and almost 10,000 operations were performed by the surgeons.

The Smiths were now planning to live most of the year in Nepal to set up the ear hospital and the rest of the year in Hereford in the UK, committing themselves to this plan by selling their house.

Meanwhile, in Surkhet, Shirley Heywood was planning a fistula centre. She was going through the planning process and also looking for funds. Her three charities were not willing to put money into buildings, at a cost of £450,000. The German agency involved with supporting the ear centre agreed to help with the fistula centre. Plans were approved, but three obstacles arose. First, the government refused to renew visas for those present more than 10 years; second, the Indian border had now been shut for several months; third, when the border opened, all supplies such as cement were much more expensive, significantly increasing the cost of the project. (The border blockade started when Nepalis of Indian heritage were unhappy with the new Nepali constitution. They sealed the main crossing points, and it appeared that the new Indian government under Prime Minister Modi was sympathetic to their cause and prevented vehicles even reaching the border. This meant severe hardship in Nepal, with huge queues for fuel, cooking gas cylinders and staple items, including medicines).

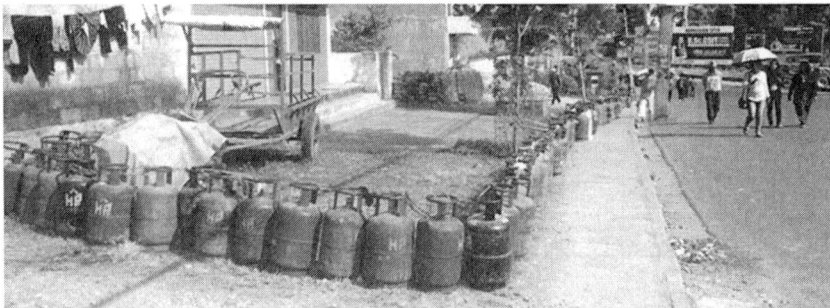

*Long lines of cooking gas bottles could be seen all around town, waiting for supplies from India.*

Following discussion with the major donors, they now required Shirley to raise 25% of the cost. Amazingly, one individual gave £100,000, and ladies in Austria, friends of Sandra Chinnery, who had worked on many gynaecology camps, were very generous. The money was found, the plans agreed, and gradually the centre, in the grounds of the main hospital in Surkhet, was built, to be opened in 2018.

In her letter of October 2014, Ellen wrote of the two camps earlier in the year where 2,500 patients were seen and 300 operations were performed. Fiona Smith, Mike's wife, joined the ear camp in Burtibang, she wrote:

"We met up with a multinational team from Australia, Germany, New Zealand and UK, a team including medical students. It lasted nine days, longer than usual. We were well fed and had hot showers. The accommodation was comfortable, unlike that of the patients, who slept on stone floors, waiting for tickets to be given out in the mornings. Many had walked for two days—just think on that. To come from so far to find help! One man had an old gunshot wound behind his ear. When this was explored, black powder was found. You don't see that every day in UK.

"The foundations are now in for the Ear Centre; the walls will soon go up." She remembered that "May and June would be very hot for the builders, and then comes the monsoon, when work can be difficult. Generally, in Pokhara, the heavy rain falls mainly at night. There are few mountain views for weeks, and at the beginning and end, violent electric storms are common. It is a very unpleasant, energy-sapping time."

The team planned for the November camps of 2014. By then, the rice had been harvested and stored, and people had more time. Two camps were planned, a gynaecology camp in Dailekh and an ear camp in Jumla. Sarah Caukwell wrote home about Dailekh: "After meeting up with the team in the Tibet Guest House hotel in Thamel, the heart of the tourist area, we went to get registered by the Nepal Medical Council. Next day's flight to Nepalganj was magnificent as we flew close to the Himalayas. From there we travelled eight hours on dodgy roads, with sheer drops all round, but as we got higher, so the views increased, and the pure mountain air was good to breathe. Dailekh is situated on a ridge, and in the mornings the valley was filled with cloud. The day started with a prayer and a thought for the day before some of us walked the 30 minutes to the hospital, such a good start." The facilities were poor, but all did well. "We asked the patients to stay in town for the 10-day duration and we checked them over. Some brought small gifts."

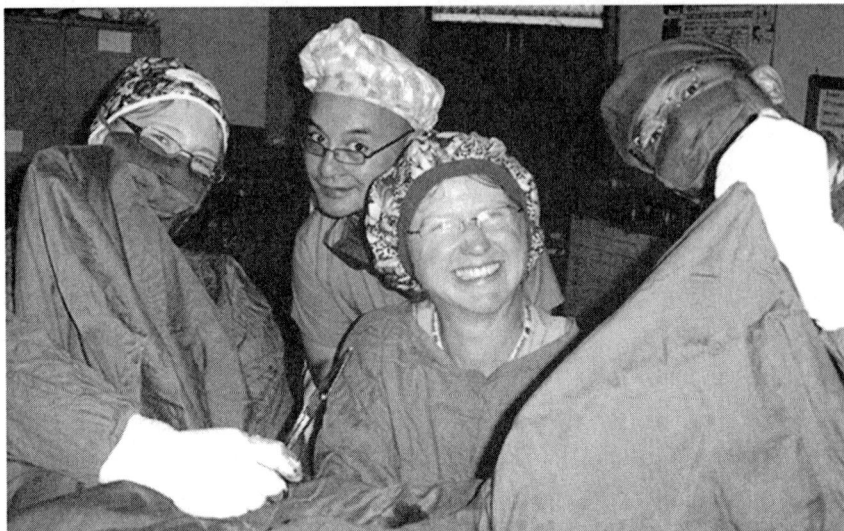

*Sarah and colleagues in the operating room.*

There was little time between these two camps, so the team was under pressure to clear up one and set up the other, with a 230-mile, 10-hour journey to face on rough, dangerous roads.

Mike Smith wrote about Jumla, the fourth ear camp at this location: "We flew from Kathmandu via Nepalganj to Jumla, with magnificent views of the hills and mountains in the clear November days. Jumla is situated in a wide valley with fabulous mountain vistas. It has a safe landing strip! Sadly the best quality flat farming land in the valley is being taken over by new concrete houses and businesses now that there is a basic road link. At an altitude of 8,000 ft, it is seriously cold in winter and can have heavy snowfall. The hospital is now well-appointed, with several specialties, including lab and X-ray facilities. The surrounding population, mostly in the hills, is about 110,000. We set up three operating tables. We quickly realised that we must get heating. Shivering surgeons are not safe, and patients on the operating table for two hours get very cold. A bottled gas heater was found.

"Trying to fit hearing aids also posed problems. The material used for the moulds didn't harden in the cold, so all fittings were done out in the sun. Work was steady and we often worked late into the evening. It is always sad to have to turn away people in need. Our ear centre will relieve that problem.

"We had been told in advance that a small girl born with no ears would be coming to see us. A company kindly donated a bone-conducting hearing aid fitted to a soft head band that would be suitable, so we brought this from England. Rare problems like this sometimes came to the camps. Providing a long-term solution is difficult, we could only try, and also inform the family of the options and support them through contact with our team in Pokhara."

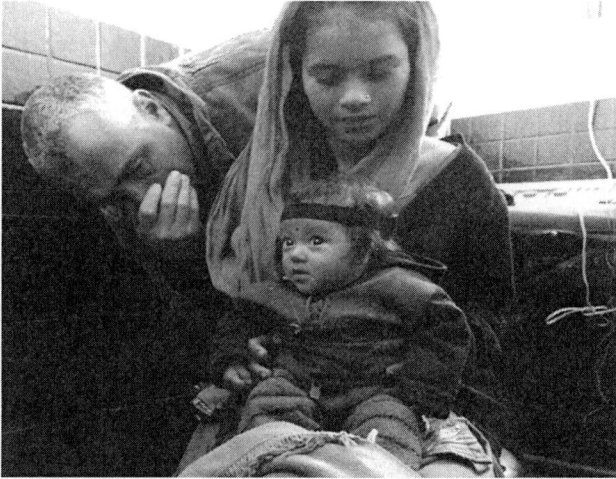

*Audiologist Phil, trials the 'softband' bone hearing aid on the small girl.*

One of Mike's anaesthetic colleagues wrote how much he enjoyed this, his second camp. He loved the flights, not only for the views, but because, on the previous trip, he had spent 14 hours in a Land Rover: "an adventure, certainly, but not one I was in a hurry to repeat! Both work and living conditions were challenging—I have rarely been colder—but it was a pleasure to work with such positive people. The basic idea is to process and treat as many patients as possible through outpatients, then operate like crazy to do the maximum possible in the limited time. The aim is to treat recurrent infections, to restore hearing and prevent the serious, even fatal complication of chronic ear disease, cholesteatoma."

This was Mike's 50th ear camp, a major landmark. He commented: "It is a huge privilege to meet the local people and hear their extraordinary stories of resilience and cheerfulness. There were many moments of fun and humour. I had the amazing experience of sitting with people in traditional dress, being for a short time part of their community, seeing a glimpse of their lives and wondering how they managed. What a chance to be given!"

The team could not have known it, but there were to be just two more camps of this type, with many expatriates. The cost and time involved in registering new doctors with the Nepal Medical Committee had become a big issue. The government then decided it did not want large groups from outside the country running medical services and stopped granting visas. The last of these camps were held in 2015, back-to-back camps in Rolpa, a surgical camp, followed by an ear camp. The camps team, after clearing up the hospital at the end of the final camp, arrived back in Pokhara after their long drive on April 25, a day which will never be forgotten in the history of Nepal.

# Chapter 22

## Earthquake

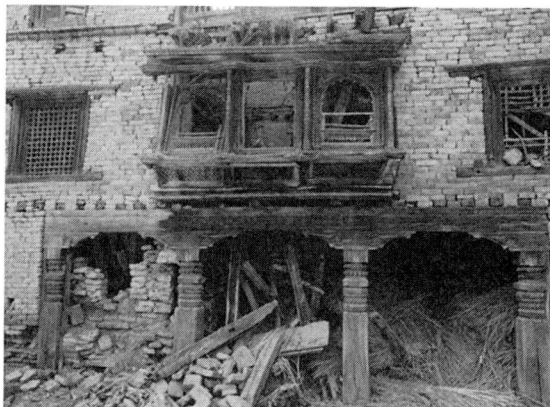

*A collapsed house near Kathmandu.*

At 11:56 am local time on 25 April 2015, a massive earthquake, with a magnitude of 7.9 on the Richter scale, struck in Gorkha District in the centre of Nepal. The destruction was massive. The UNESCO World Heritage site in Kathmandu was severely damaged. Fortunately, it was a Saturday, so offices and schools were empty, and in the villages, people would be in their fields, thereby reducing the death toll. Nevertheless, it was said that 10,000 people were killed and 22,000 injured. Many houses and buildings were destroyed, and people made homeless.

There were aftershocks every 20 minutes. Rescue groups later brought in many tents and some senior politicians chose to sleep outdoors. The large parade ground, the Tundikhel, in the centre of Kathmandu, was covered with tents for weeks as people sought a safe shelter. Thankfully, the weather was warm. Mt Everest had its most deadly day as a huge avalanche killed 21 people, and the base camp, busy in this climbing season, needed evacuating. It was days before a helicopter approached the epicentre. It was a devastating experience.

Yet Pokhara, as near the epicentre as Kathmandu, felt the earth shake but little damage was done. Mike, who had returned to Pokhara after camp, planned to travel on home the next day. He was standing outside the ear centre, checking building progress. "We saw buildings sway and felt the earth jumping, the ground continued to vibrate for some hours, with occasional aftershocks." The ear centre only suffered minor cracks in the plaster; it had been built deliberately single-storied and on a double concrete slab, with walls following earthquake resistant techniques.

Nepal had been overdue a major quake for some years. All the destructive force went to the east. That meant that Pokhara would, for months, even years, become a vital centre for rescue and then rebuilding shattered homes and lives. INF found itself a crucial aid donor, and acted quickly through its network of offices, friends and donors, in countries such as the UK, Australia and New Zealand, to send practical help. They rapidly contacted all the camps and INF staff and informed their families that they were safe. Plans for subsequent medical camps were abandoned and all available help put into the rescue effort, including the camps team and vehicles.

The team immediately repacked the truck and headed off towards Gorkha, with little information about the situation there. One of the Nepali team member's own family lived in the area which turned out to be the epicentre. They were the first agency to reach that affected area and bring help. The monsoon was but six weeks away and people needed shelter. Later, the government required all aid money to be directed through it. The idea of centralising the rescue programme was good, but the government couldn't handle it efficiently; it was too under-resourced to use it quickly and some was left unused, or 'wasted' who knows where. A spin-off from these terrible events was that INF set up a disaster response and recovery team.

Some returning camp volunteers were actually on the tarmac leaving Kathmandu when the quake struck. The pilot saw something was happening to the airfield and took off. Mike, travelling a day later, passed many collapsed buildings on the road into Kathmandu. People were standing stunned, outside in the open. He shared a hotel room with a climber, evacuated injured from Everest. After a few aftershocks and despite the rain, Mike went and slept in the hotel garden. He then spent 24 hours in the departure lounge at the airport, as big transport planes arrived with rescue teams, dogs and supplies from around the world. But there was so little information about where the rescue teams were needed that they had to sit and wait. Tourists had to be flown home; there was a big backlog. The airport, though damaged, was useable and relief flights remained the priority, not passenger planes. The main tourist area around Thamel was badly damaged. There were enormous tensions. Another quake on May 12 was 6.3 strength, frightening locals and adding to the damage to unstable buildings. For weeks, many in Kathmandu slept out under tarpaulins. It took time before the devastation and death toll in some mountain villages became evident.

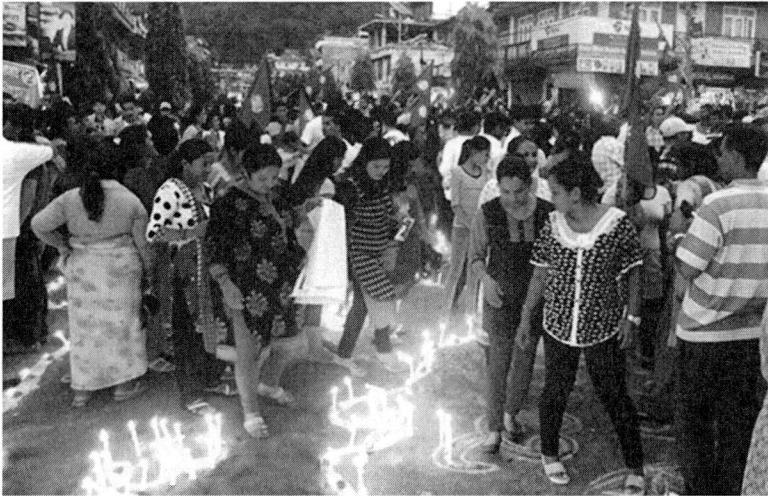

*The long-awaited new constitution was greeted with celebrations in Pokhara, but within days, dissatisfaction was evident across the country.*

Later that year, the tribal people on the Nepali side of the Indian border rose up again, unhappy with the new constitution, which divided the country into provinces, partly along ethnic and language lines. Those areas in the plains were very little damaged by the earthquakes. There are many unknowns in all this. Whatever the cause, the Nepal/India border was again closed. Kathmandu and Pokhara were particularly hard hit. No fuel, long queues, no bottled gas or kerosene for cooking, none of the vast array of Indian fruit and vegetables. No building materials. It was a very effective, damaging blockade, at a time critical for the rebuilding of Nepal. It went on for months.

The 'black market' thrived. Eventually there was a political settlement and life slowly returned, not to normal, but to caring for the dispossessed. Years later, many in quake affected areas still lived in temporary shelters, schools functioning as best they could without proper buildings. The closing of the border and prevention of supplies coming by land through India was a severe handicap, and it is hard to understand why it was allowed.

# Chapter 23

## The Ear Hospital

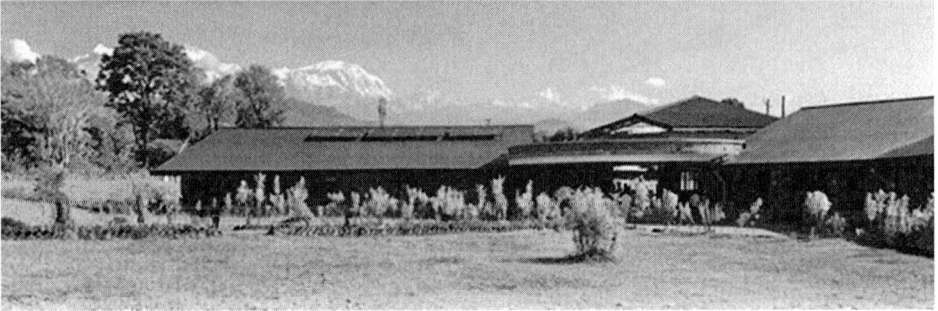

*The Ear Centre, at Green Pastures Hospital, with Annapurna mountains.*

"The Ear Hospital and Training Centre is up and running!" To quote Mike and Fiona: "The ear hospital is a triumph! It is a very happy place to work in, and the new staff are settling in and being well looked after by the camps team. The engineers have completed an amazing building, on time and under budget."

Mike had first sketched the hospital layout on the back of an envelope, then discussed the flow of patients and overall layout with medical colleagues and asked an old friend who was an architect to draw plans. Then they added services like piped oxygen and air conditioning for the operating theatre. This was then taken to a Nepali architectural firm for detailed plans, and finally, a local contractor was appointed. INF engineers oversaw the building as it progressed, ensuring the quality of materials and the project management were correct. Mike expressed some worries: "The recent India/Nepal border closure has meant that our container of equipment was still being held in Calcutta after several months. Sadly, due to a catalogue of difficulties, the container never reached Pokhara. This was a terrible loss, as a generous donor had covered the costs. It was painful to explain to her. Eka Dev and I have searched high and low, but it has been difficult to obtain all the furniture and fittings for the hospital, we drew up designs and local carpenters made what was needed. The petrol shortage has also made it difficult for people from the far west to get to the hospital."

Again, there were delays in obtaining work visas. Posts for experts had been approved by the government and projects were Nepali led, but delays meant that visas expired, then the limited periods allowed on tourist visas also ran out. Fortunately for the INF projects, Nepalis had now been in place for some years as project heads, so the projects continued. There was great uncertainty among the expatriate community. For INF families, when their existing visa ran out and they returned home, possibly at a bad time for the schooling of any children involved, it meant that there was no certainty that they would ever get a visa again. The disruption for families was severe. Mike and Fiona Smith were also caught up in this problem. They could not return to the hospital for many months. The government had made it clear that a person could not return on a tourist visa and work. Fortunately, two young Nepali surgeons had joined the team and were able to do assessments and some surgery but needed an experienced surgeon to teach them and improve their range and techniques. It was a very frustrating stand-off.

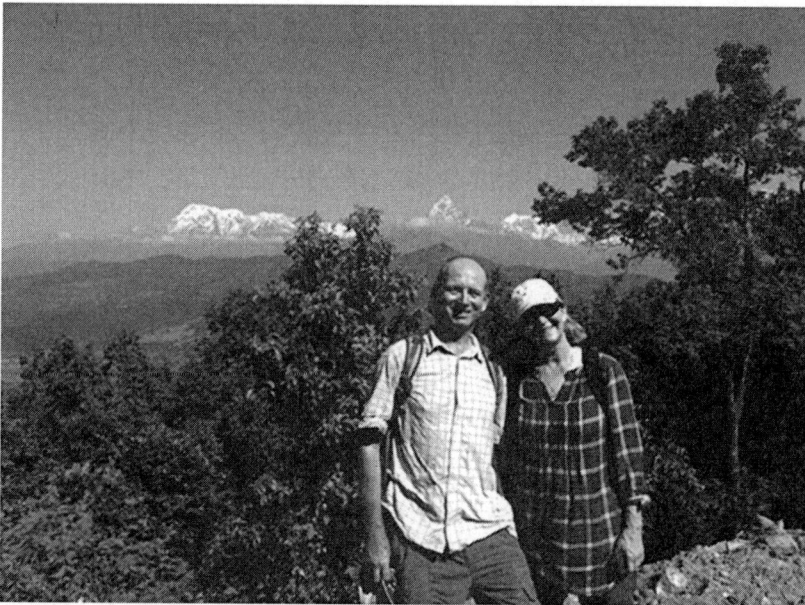

*Mike and Fiona in Pokhara, with the famous Machhapuchare peak (Fishtail) and the Annapurna mountain range.*

In other respects, the timing for an ear centre was excellent. Roads were being built and existing roads improved. A highway is planned through the 'middle hills', which will make access easier for people in the northern districts to reach Pokhara and Kathmandu. The need for ear camps in the remote hills is less and resources can be concentrated. There is a plan to run ear outreach screening and health education visits, after training paramedical staff.

The site is excellent, within the grounds and part of Green Pastures Hospital, one mile from the main bus station and little more from the airport, which it overlooks. The climate for eight months of the year is pleasant, the view of seven peaks over 26,000 ft is magnificent. How wonderful that this site, once rejected by the local people because it had been occupied by a leprosarium, was now providing an excellent home for several vital social and medical specialties, especially those which were poorly catered for elsewhere in the west of the country.

The UK charity, Ear Aid Nepal has progressed from supporting ear camps and advising volunteers, to offering annual training bursaries, to enable young Nepali ear surgeons and audiologists to attend courses and conferences outside Nepal. It funds training courses for Ear Centre staff, and some scholarships to enable young British surgeons to visit Nepal, take part in the work and lead educational seminars. EAN also works with international academic institutions, participating in research projects. It has helped provide equipment and is a major funder of care for ear patients unable to contribute towards their medical costs.

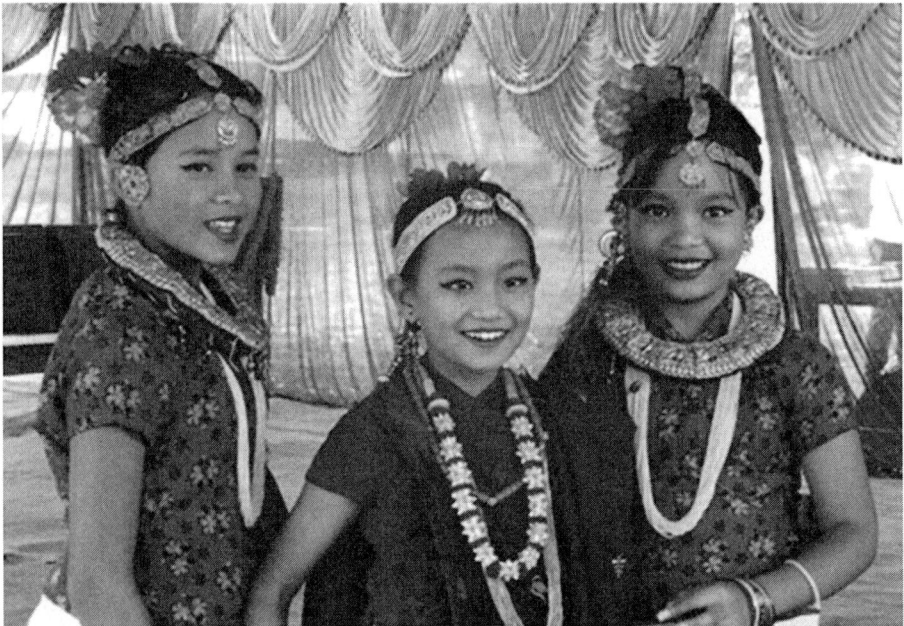

*Traditionally dressed girls danced at the opening ceremony.*

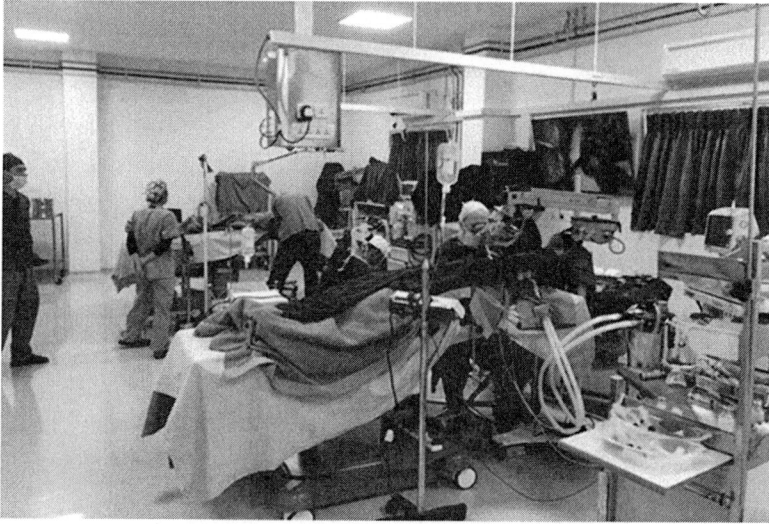

*The operating room at the new Ear Centre.*

Mike returned to Nepal, to continue giving treatment and training, until the Coronavirus outbreak forced him to leave in 2020, on one of the last planes allowed out from Kathmandu. Just prior to his leaving, the first cochlear implant to be performed in Nepal outside Kathmandu, by a Nepali surgeon, took place in the Ear Centre. How incredible to witness the facilities being used by experienced and talented local surgeons.

In 2018, the fistula hospital was finally opened, inspired by the observed needs of women attending the medical camps. Fully equipped, in the grounds of the government hospital in Surkhet, it would provide fistula repair work in an ideal situation. The plan was to operate on five patients a week, 250 a year. Small scale, Nepali-led gynaecology camps continued on an occasional basis. Long-term, the hope must be that good midwifery care throughout Nepal would make fistulas a thing of the past.

Late in 2019, Ellen Findlay returned briefly to Nepal. For some years, she had looked after the finances of a former colleague, Eileen Lodge who, with another nurse, Betty Bailey, had founded the leprosy project in 1954 and established the work at Green Pastures Hospital, which opened in 1957. In 1970, Eileen left Pokhara to establish a new community for leprosy sufferers, rejected by their own families. On her way to Kathmandu, changing planes at Bhairahawa, on the Indian border, she met Ellen, who had just arrived in Nepal for the first time from the port of Mumbai. They spoke briefly before Ellen flew the 20 minutes to Pokhara, and Eileen flew to Kathmandu. They remained friends till Eileen died.

Eileen set up home in Kathmandu, where she opened a leatherwork and craft rehabilitation centre to provide work for those needing help. Faced with the plight of many ex-leprosy patients, she continued to set up new communities for them in Lalgardh (where she established the Nepal Leprosy Trust) and elsewhere in the Terai. She had taken Nepali citizenship, relinquishing her UK passport. She returned, finally, to live in Kathmandu, latterly cared for by her Nepali 'family', until her death, aged 94. Ellen, named as her next-of-kin, returned to Nepal to take care of her affairs. She had very little: a cooker, a fridge, a washing machine, a bed and a chair, all now given to her Nepali family.

Eileen's funeral was attended by a large crowd in Kathmandu, and her body was then taken on the six-hour journey to Green Pastures, in Pokhara, now expanded to include one of Nepal's first centres for palliative care, in addition to the leprosy and ear centres and the spinal rehabilitation centre. There, after a memorable service, the first in the newly built multipurpose learning centre, Eileen was laid to rest, in the place of her vision, near the site of her original grass-roofed home and clinic. [2] Many of those attending had been her patients or colleagues, and there were emotional moments of shared memories.

Ellen had worked there 40 years before, and her work in Nepal was now completed, 50 years after she had arrived off that long sea and rail journey via Mumbai. People used to ask her: "What will happen to camps when you are not here?" Her reply? "If it is God's work, it will continue." As Hudson Taylor said, "God's work, done in God's way will not lack God's resources." "Camps are not mine." said Ellen, "It is God's work, and He will bring it to an end in His time. I must say, I was not surprised when the Nepali government made so many restrictions, and it was impossible for us to continue camps as we had known them. We are grateful for the many lives that were touched. The lasting legacy of camps is the people who would otherwise never have had surgery or treatment for various conditions and those who received training. Green Pastures Hospital continues that work in new ways."

---

[2] The story of Eileen's work can be read in *A Touch of Providence*. NLT (www.nlt.org.uk)

# Appendix 1

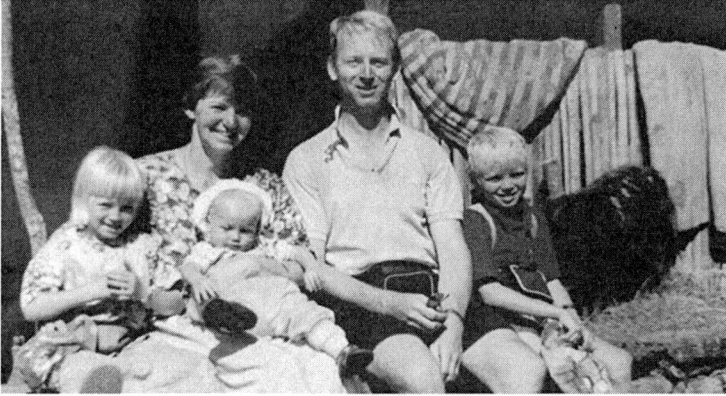

*The Smiths trekking in 1992*
*Lydia, Fiona, Abigail, Mike and Luke.*

Dr Mike Smith tells his story:

People often ask, "Why do you do this, you must love Nepal?" Yes, but that is only part of the story and a complete answer would have to include faith, adventure, and the opportunity to use skills. At medical school, I took up outdoor sports, like white water canoeing and rock climbing. When the opportunity for a student elective in India came along, I went. That was a wake-up call, arriving in Mumbai in the spring, travelling overland to Chennai, then on to Vellore Christian Medical College to study, but quickly taking chances to travel to Sri Lanka and to Nepal, in the May heat. Amid all the excitement and colour, I saw real poverty and was shocked. Some impressive people tried to interest me in Christian faith, including a lady missionary who had run a clinic in the middle of India for many years and was having treatment for terminal cancer, and a young Indian man who persuaded me to take a Gideon's new testament Bible. But I had no experience of church and I did not take an interest.

Back at Medical school I was offered a lift to North Wales to go climbing in Snowdonia with members of the college Christian Union. What I had not expected was that we would go to Beddgelert church, or that a young blind man would speak and hold my attention. As I remember it, he spoke about sin and our need for trust in Jesus. How he 'knocks at the door' and will enter our lives and change them if we allow Him. At the time I felt very annoyed that his words had jolted me. It was made more complicated because I fell for Fiona, who was one of the Christians on the trip. I started to read and question. A friend gave me a modern Bible translation and said I should read the book of John. I had to admit that it sounded genuine, as John wrote of his experiences. I read a lot of books, notably Mere Christianity by C S Lewis and Basic Christianity by John Stott, demonstrating the uniqueness and the historical evidence for Jesus. I quizzed people, I read about other major religions, and I attended some church meetings.

During this time, I flew to Pakistan, travelled alone overland to Nepal and trekked to Everest. Randomly I picked up a book from a trolley on an Indian railway station, it was "The Life of Jesus Christ" by Lord Longford, summarising the four gospels. Then, when trekking, I walked much of the way with another lone trekker, who was reading a paperback copy of the New Testament. We were both curious, and discussed it. I got to the point where I had an intellectual understanding and even belief that Jesus had existed and that, as C S Lewis famously said, "He had to be mad, bad or God", and only the last made sense. Then I was stuck with this knowledge and what to do next, until I talked to Fiona's church pastor. Bill pointed me to a Bible verse: "If anyone acknowledges that Jesus is the Son of God, God lives in him and he in God." (1 John 4, v 15). Bill showed me that I had already intellectually accepted the truth but needed to open the door and simply trust and ask Jesus to take me on. We knelt and I prayed. Something happened that evening which changed me. Our friends saw it, and no one questioned the change, (for the better!)

Fiona, who had trained as a physio, and I decided to offer whatever talents we had to Christian service overseas. I wrote to several groups working in various continents, and had a personal reply from INF. They needed a doctor to work in the leprosy hospital at Green Pastures and suggested that we, a newly married couple, should go to Nepal for two years, to work and learn some language. I had started training as an ENT surgeon and this was a big change in direction. In 1980 we went to Ethiopia for leprosy training, then straight on to Nepal, where we went through many exciting and difficult experiences. On returning to England, I completed ENT training. Then in 1990, we returned to Nepal with our two young children (Luke and Lydia) and set up an ENT department in the regional hospital. Our third child (Abigail) was born there. After eight years, I took a consultant post in Hereford and Worcester in England, but continued to arrange camps, and travelled frequently to Nepal. It was busy juggling these two jobs, but worth every minute. It was sometimes hard to travel yet again, but once we reached a village and saw the patients, the culture and the scenery, the tiredness disappeared. It was great to have new groups of volunteers, old friends, colleagues and supporters, focused on doing everything they could to help. But behind all this was prayer. Developing the Ear Centre and continuing the camps was a big challenge. Without belief and the strength that came from following that call to serve, we could not have continued. Jesus says, "If you remain in me and I in you, you will bear much fruit; apart from me you can do nothing." (John 15,5).

# Appendix 2 by Dr Mike Smith

## The Anatomy, Pathology and Surgery of the Ear

Each ear is normally described in three anatomical parts: the outer ear, middle ear and inner ear. The interpretation of incoming sounds by various parts of the brain is also vital. The processing, in the brain, of the sound signals coming from the ears, enables us to distinguish different sounds in noise or be alert to danger or a child's call, when we are listening to something else. It also lets us discriminate and interpret the multitude of frequencies of sound, even in normal speech, into words that make sense of the language we understand. Have you noticed how you can recognise someone mentioning your name, even in a crowd of people? When we walk through a forest and hear a twig snap or a deer cough, or we are crossing the road, or talking to a group of friends at a party, we need to know which direction sound comes from. The slight delay between sounds reaching our two ears enables us to do this. Hearing is a very complex process, and we are only just starting to understand it.

The ears have more than one function; they are also important for balance and position sense. If you suffer from travel or seasickness or hate the rides at fairgrounds, then you know what happens when the balance apparatus in our ears is disturbed or confused.

The outer ear is composed of the eardrum, the ear canal and the visible part on the outside of the head, which is called the pinna or the auricle. The pinna helps to collect sounds and funnel them into the ear canal. When a dog or a horse pricks its ears, it is using small muscles around the ear to move the pinna and focus on the direction of the sound to localise it accurately. We also have these muscles and some people can wiggle their ears, but the benefit is limited in humans. Although we do not move our ears much, we do use the funnelling effect of the pinna, and we turn our heads to help us decide the direction of the sound. The ear canal is about 2.5cm long in an adult and has a gentle S shape. This is protective, so that straight objects cannot easily reach the eardrum and damage it. The outer part of the ear canal has small hairs and also glands that make waxy secretions. All of these are designed to protect the canal. The wax has several important functions: it makes the skin flexible and waterproof, and it has antiseptic properties. Importantly, the skin in the ear canal grows very slowly in an outward direction which carries dead skin flakes, hairs and wax outwards. This also carries with it dust, sand etc. that may have entered the ear. So the ear has a self-cleansing mechanism, and that is why we do not normally need to clean inside our ears. Attempts to do so, or the use of hearing aids, tend to push that wax back into the ear, where it accumulates and may become obstructive. It is only once wax completely blocks the ear canal that it significantly affects hearing. The normal eardrum is a thin but quite robust membrane about the size of your small fingernail. It moves in and out with the vibrations of sound in the air, or with other sudden air pressure changes.

The middle ear is a small space, normally containing air and the three small bones of hearing (the ossicles). We have three ossicles in each ear: the Malleus bone (hammer shaped), the Incus (anvil shaped) and the smallest bone in the human body, the Stapes bone (which looks like a stirrup on a horse's saddle). These bones link the eardrum (the tympanic membrane) to the inner ear. When these bones or the eardrum are damaged or absent it causes a 'conductive' hearing loss. That is, the sound vibrations are not transmitted effectively from the air outside into the fluids of the inner ear. Infections often damage this system.

The inner ear consists of some small tunnels inside the bone, deep in the ear. This bone forms part of the bottom of the skull and is called the petrous bone. It is the hardest bone in the body; it is like rock (which is what petrous means). These tunnels (the labyrinth) have two main parts. The cochlea, which is a coiled tube a bit like a snail shell in shape contains the nerve endings that detect the movements of the eardrum and send information to the brain about loudness and pitch of sounds. It is quite incredible that we can discern so many different sounds simultaneously, across a wide range of pitches. Unfortunately, this range diminishes with age because the nerve endings (hair cells) slowly deteriorate. Some animals have much more range, but we have the advantage of more brain processing power, complex language and speech skills. When the inner ear or the nerves connected to it are damaged then we call this a nerve deafness (or 'sensorineural' hearing loss). In many people affected by chronic ear infections, they will have both conductive and sensorineural ('mixed' type) hearing loss.

In Nepal, we see all forms of hearing loss at higher incidences than occur in most more-developed countries. The reasons are varied. For example, there is a

199

lower rate of vaccination, so infections such as measles, mumps, rubella and meningitis, which can all cause hearing loss, are more common. Ear infections such as acute otitis media, which are common in small children everywhere but usually settle with few if any complications in countries with better healthcare, are commoner and lead to worse outcomes. Infections like this in Nepal often go on to cause permanent large perforations of the eardrums and also infection in the mastoid bone behind the ear. It seems that some races are a little more prone to these problems perhaps due to variations in skull shape, and these infections are also related to poverty and poor living standards.

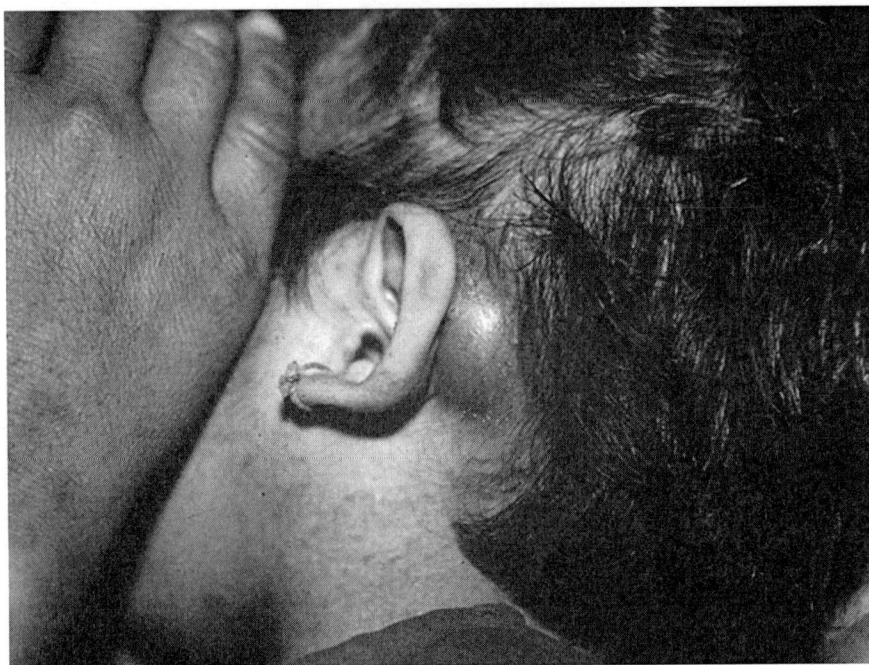

*A young boy with an acute mastoid abscess.*

Living in a smoke or dust-filled home or environment may well aggravate the problem. As living conditions improve, it is likely that ear diseases caused by infection will become less common in the future. However, other problems such as noise-induced hearing loss are increasing due to industrialisation, without adequate health and safety precautions. Nepalis also seem to love huge loudspeakers and microphones at social gatherings!

Sometimes ear infection spreads and causes serious complications such as mastoid abscess, meningitis or brain abscesses, which can be fatal.

Balance is the other important function of the ears. There are two main types of balance organ in each ear, one part mainly detects head position, and the other part detects direction or change in speed of head movement. When we stand still or turn quickly, we are using these systems to allow our brain to control other things such as fixing our eyes on an object. This is needed whenever we move our head or when we trip unexpectedly and put out a hand or leg to steady us. The sense of balance is often forgotten when we think of our usual five senses, but it is critical. Think of a gymnast or ballet dancer, who needs an extremely good sense of balance. This sense is also vital in our simplest movements, such as walking or standing on a moving bus. When this sense is damaged we can experience falls or dizziness (vertigo), both of which can be very distressing or dangerous.

The ear also contains other important structures, which can be prone to damage with some infections or injuries, in particular, the facial nerve. This nerve controls all our movements of facial expression such as smiling, frowning, whistling and closing our eyes. If this nerve is paralysed or weak, we cannot protect our eyes from injury, we dribble, and our face looks quite disfigured and crooked.

There are many diseases and problems that can affect the ear. Many are preventable, but once established, we also have a wide range of possible treatments. Amongst these is surgery. In Nepal, middle ear and mastoid infection is very common and can affect any age group, though often the most severe cases are found in children. We usually have three aims with this type of surgery. Firstly, we want to remove infected tissue and stop further extension and complications; secondly, we hope to achieve a dry, non-discharging ear; and thirdly, we do our best to restore hearing, either by the surgery or by hearing aids, once infection has resolved.

Common operations are myringoplasty and tympanoplasty. Without going into technical details, these are operations to repair perforations or damage of the eardrum. It is immensely satisfying to repair the eardrums of a child when they have big holes in the drums of both ears and suffer marked conductive deafness. We know that by a relatively simple operation, we can stop the ear discharge and enable a return to school and education. To these surgeries we often add ossiculoplasty at the same time. This means that we repair ossicle bones in the middle ear that have been eroded by infection, to try and restore hearing. We can either use the patient's own tissues such as bone grafts from elsewhere in the ear or we can use a range of artificial materials such as titanium implants. These implants are expensive and sometimes work their way out of the eardrum over the years, so we prefer to use the patient's own tissue whenever possible. We have had to learn to sculpt tiny bones and fit them accurately. Whilst not always effective, this can work well and is certainly worth attempting in an environment like Nepal where hearing aids, repairs and the batteries can be expensive or impractical for patients. This is particularly true for economically poorer patients and those from remote areas.

Sometimes the infection has spread into the mastoid bone (especially in a common condition called cholesteatoma). This has to be cleared very carefully in order to reduce the chance of recurrence. There are many types of mastoidectomy needed, and they depend on the extent of spread of the disease. We encounter very extensive disease in Nepal because treatment is often late. Some of the patients have infected holes (fistulae) or scars behind the ear due to multiple abscesses. It is beyond imagining what pain these people (often children) must have gone through over the years. Very skilled surgery is required for these patients in order to remove disease and restore some function. The disease often affects both ears, and they need staged procedures to correct both sides.

There are many other variations and types of ear surgery used for different conditions; this is just a brief overview. Everything in the ear is very small, so we do most of our work through an operating microscope for magnification. We are also starting to do 'keyhole' endoscopic ear surgery using small telescopes in the ear canal, whilst watching on a video screen.

# Appendix 3
## Further Information

The International Nepal Fellowship continues to support the disadvantaged in western Nepal, through health and community programmes based in centres such as Pokhara, Nepalganj and Surkhet, and many more remote, rural locations.
INF also has country offices in Nepal, the UK, USA, Canada, Australia and New Zealand, and links to other international organisations assisting the work. More details are available on the following websites:

INF: https://www.inf.org

Ear Aid Nepal: https://www.earaidnepal.org

Also by David Hawker:

Kanchi Doctor: Ruth Watson of Nepal

A Week in August: 70 Years of Changing Lives at a School Christian Camp

Author's contact: dh11141@yahoo.co.uk